SRN 2 REVISION BOOK

CASE STUDIES AND OBJECTIVE TEST QUESTIONS

Edited and compiled by
LYNN COPCUTT SRN DN(London) RNT. B.Ed.(Hons).
Senior Tutor, Queen Elizabeth School of Nursing,
Edgbaston, Birmingham.

PASTEST SERVICE
Hemel Hempstead
Hertfordshire England

P.O. Box 81, Hemel Hempstead, Hertfordshire

First published 1983

ISBN 0-906896-09-6

British Library Cataloguing in Publication Data

Copcutt, Lynn
SRN 2 : case histories and objective test questions for student nurses.
1. Nursing - Problems, exercises, etc.
I. Title
610'73'076 RT55

ISBN 0-906896-09-6

Text prepared using Sirius 1 microcomputer.
Phototypeset by Designed Publications using an interface.
Printed by Martins of Berwick.

CONTENTS

Brackets indicate the number of case studies in each subject.
Each case study has 4 related questions.

NOTES TO THE READER

This book has been produced to assist student nurses preparing for the multiple choice paper of the State Final Examination for the General Register, established by the General Nursing Council for England and Wales.

All examinations create anxiety for candidates. Multiple choice questions can pose particular difficulties for some people either because of lack of experience in attempting this type of test, or because previously they have been faced with questions which bear little similarity to those found in the actual examination. I therefore feel there is a need for this book and its sister edition for pupil nurses, because they contain carefully selected, pre-tested and validated questions specifically intended to prepare the learner nurse for the amended GNC State Final Examination which begins in January 1983.

Practising nurse teachers were invited to submit questions for consideration. Over 250 case studies were scrutinized to obtain the 52 finally accepted. After initial editing the questions were compiled into test papers of approximately 100 questions each. These tests were then taken by a minimum of 100 finalist student nurses in more than 60 schools of nursing throughout the country.

Computer analysis followed and only those questions meeting predetermined levels of difficulty and discrimination were considered for inclusion. In addition, comments received from student nurses and teaching staff participating with the pre-testing of questions were considered. Thank-you all for your co-operation.

The preparation of multiple choice tests is not easy, but every attempt has been made to ensure that this publication will become a helpful part of the arduous task of examination revision.

This book contains 240 multiple choice questions, 180 of which are compiled into 45 case studies each with 4 questions. The remaining 60 questions are grouped together as a practice examination consisting of 7 case studies and 32 individual questions, grouped together in order to cover the range of topics and degree of difficulty the student is likely to meet.

Each question consists of an initial statement followed by four alternative answers, marked A B C D. Only *one* of these is correct.

Questions are printed on the right-hand page, with the correct answers and explanations on the following page. Alongside each answer you will find a percentage figure which indicates the number of finalist nurses who chose the correct answer during pre-testing of the questions. Questions with a high percentage are easier than those with a low percentage. By using this information you will be able to identify areas which need concentrated revision. It will also enable you to assess your own level of performance relative to that of other finalists. Attempt each question before you look at the answers, this is the best way to test your knowledge and to highlight strengths and weaknesses.

Finally, a word of thanks to the many people who have assisted with the preparation of this book, especially the teachers who wrote initial questions and answers for editing, the student nurses and their teachers who co-operated so willingly with the pre-testing, and to my own students whose advice and criticisms were invaluable.

I am most grateful to you all.

L.C.

WHAT IS A MULTIPLE CHOICE QUESTION?

A multiple choice question consists of a "stem" and several alternative options. The stem is the part which states the nursing problem and poses the question. In the GNC multiple choice questions there are four alternative answers marked A, B, C, and D. Only ***one*** answer in each set of four alternatives is correct, the other three are all incorrect and are therefore known as distractors, i.e. their purpose is to attempt to distract the candidate from the correct answer.

e.g Which one of the following describes hyperchromic macrocytic red cells:

A. Small cells with high haemoglobin content
B. Large cells with low haemoglobin content
C. Small cells with low haemoglobin content
D. Large cells with high haemoglobin content

A, B, and C, are distractors
D is the correct answer.

WHY A MULTIPLE CHOICE EXAMINATION?

1. ***Because a large part of the syllabus can be included.***

   In the GNC Afternoon Examination paper of 60 multiple choice questions many aspects of the syllabus can be tested, therefore do not panic if on looking at the questions there are some that you simply cannot do. Very few people if any, sitting the same examination as you will be able to answer every question correctly. Remember that you can afford to get a good many wrong and still pass the examination.

2. ***Because it is possible to test more than just memory and rote learning.***

   By far the greatest emphasis in the examination is on ***thinking*** and ***reasoning,*** so do not dash off your answers quickly. The time allowed, 1 ½ hours, is deliberately very generous giving candidates plenty of time to sit and think and to work out their answers logically and systematically, so ***do not worry*** if at first glance the questions appear complex for you will have lots of time to clarify your thoughts. Calm down and take one question at a time.

e.g Which one of the following groups of pathways will be followed by an upper motor neurone serving the right side of the body:

A left motor cortex, left lateral tract of spinal cord, right anterior horn cell
B right motor cortex, left lateral tract of spinal cord,left anterior horn cell
C left motor cortex, right lateral tract of spinal cord, right anterior horn cell
D right motor cortex, right lateral tract of spinal cord, left anterior horn cell.

In order to work out the correct answer to this rather nasty question:

1. Stay calm; do not panic.
2. Read the stem again carefully. What clues are there? Note that the motor neurone serves the ***right*** side of the body. So, it must originate in the left motor cortex of the brain.
3. Check the 4 options and cross out any that include right motor cortex.
4. Check the remaining 2 options A and C. Note that both include "right anterior horn cell" so this can be accepted as correct information. Option A includes "left lateral tract of spinal cord" but Option C includes "right lateral tract of spinal cord"
5. Using your knowledge of the nervous system you can work out that C is correct, (remember that motor pathways ***cross over*** at the base of the brain).

   i.e. left motor cortex
   right lateral tract of spinal cord
   right anterior horn cell

3. *Because candidates can be tested on their ability to evaluate.*

The "best" course of action or "most" important priority, the "immediate" first aid treatment or "first" action may be asked for. In such questions as these it can be difficult to differentiate between the four alternatives offered for they may all seem to be a possible correct response. When this happens, go back to the beginning of the question and re-read it slowly, deliberately looking for any clues given in the wording.

e.g. Which one of the following would be ***most*** effective when helping a new patient settle in to a long stay ward for elderly patients:

A leave her to settle in gradually in her own time
B talk to her frequently of family and home
C encourage her to join in ward activities
D ensure she can see the television from her chair

A, B, and D are distractors, although each could perhaps contribute to the initial reaction to admission. However C is correct because of the 4 options this would ***most*** assist the "settling in" process.

4. ***Because all multiple choice questions can be pre-tested.***

Multiple choice questions are distributed to finalist nurses in Schools of Nursing across the country in order to discover how easy or difficult each question is and to eliminate any poor questions. When the State Final multiple choice paper is set, each question's degree of difficulty is known, and therefore a fair mix of questions can be given in every examination. Whenever you sit your GNC Multiple Choice Examination, overall it should not be much easier or harder than any previous examination. Pre-testing also means that very hard or very easy questions can be omitted, but be prepared for the fact that there will be very few questions that you will know the answer to immediately without some thought and working out. Be reassured that every other candidate in the country is in the same position.

5. ***Because any examiner bias, when marking the answers, is eliminated.***

Handwriting, spelling, grammar and examiner preferences for specialist subjects cannot in any way influence the result since each question has only one correct answer and the examination sheet is computer marked.

NOTES FOR GENERAL GUIDANCE

1. In the General Nursing Council Examination the multiple choice questions are printed in booklet form with about 8 questions to the page. Be prepared for the fact that the print is fairly small, sometimes this comes as rather a surprise to candidates and is enough initially to jar their concentration.

2. Choose whichever of the four distractors you feel is correct and do not worry or be put off if you seem to have, for example, four "B" correct answers in a row. This is perfectly possible, have the courage of your convictions.

3. Remember that you can change your mind and alter your answer on the computer sheet. However, having done this it is ***impossible*** to return to your original choice of answer. So think carefully before committing yourself. Once done, leave that question and move on to the next.

4. When revising do not just sit passively reading books and lecture notes, but remember that many multiple choice questions will test your ability to reason. Therefore, when revising, try to understand ***why*** nursing care and observations are carried out, and their significance.
   Questions which test your ability to reason or your understanding of nursing care could ask:

   > Which one of the following is the *reason* why a patient with chronic bronchitis is prescribed a low-concentration of oxygen?

   or

   > A patient with dyspnoea is nursed in the upright position ***because.......***

   A question testing your memory only could be as follows:

   > Which of the following patients rely on a lowered oxygen level in order to stimulate respiration? The patient suffering from
   >
   > A pneumonia
   > B chronic bronchitis
   > C pneumothorax
   > D bronchiectasis

   When revising, instead of saying to yourself "the patient following cholecystectomy will need chest physiotherapy" you ought really to be asking yourself "why does the patient following cholecystectomy need chest physiotherapy?". Similarly, instead of "the patient with hypertension may need renal investigations" try "why does the hypertensive patient need renal investigations?". This will give an added depth to your revision and will most certainly enhance your chances of success in the multiple choice examination.

Here are some more examples of revision questions:

> Why does the patient with pneumonia complain of pain on inspiration?
> Why does constipation predispose to the development of diverticular disease?
> Why is a high protein diet prescribed for a patient with nephrotic syndrome?
> Why is a t-tube clamped prior to removal?
> Why, if the victim is shocked, should a light cover only be used at the scene of an accident?
> Why does albuminuria contribute to the formation of oedema?
> Why do patients need bed- rest following a myocardial infarction?
> Why is oxygen humidified?

5. If all else fails and you simply cannot work out the correct answer to any particular question ***always*** attempt the question and choose one of the four alternatives. Marks are not deducted for wrong answers therefore you have nothing to lose.
   In the Final Examination ***always attempt every question.***

6. Work methodically through the test reading only ***one*** question at a time. Try to work out the answer but if you cannot, ***leave a space*** on the computer answer sheet and move on to the next question.

7. Check carefully throughout the test that you are marking your answer in the correct space on the computer answer sheet.

8. Having worked through the test once, return to questions you left earlier and attempt to answer them. If all else fails, guess!

9. On completion of the test, check that your candidate number is entered correctly and leave. It is not generally advisable to go back to the beginning of the test checking every answer as this could cause you to make rushed last minute alterations which cannot then be re-corrected.

10. If you can, avoid the temptation to discuss your answers with your colleagues afterwards since this will add to your anxiety. Questions are seldom remembered accurately, so it is far better to wait patiently for results day!

Good Luck.

REVISION GUIDE

The following checklist is intended to help you structure and plan your revision effectively, although the list is by no means complete.

Try to adopt a "total care" approach using the following master plan. It can be applied to any patient care situation and encompasses both drug therapy and nursing observations, as well as community and hospital based management.

Relate physiology to the signs and symptoms as you work through each list of disorders, rather than try to master each independently.

MASTER PLAN

Identify patient problems for each topic in the revision guide:

1) Physical problems
2) Social problems
3) Emotional problems

Remember that problems can be ***actual*** (existing) or ***potential*** (likely to arise unless deliberately prevented) in each of the 3 categories above.

Additionally, when considering patient problems the following checklist may be a useful starting point:

Maintaining a safe environment
Communicating
Personal cleanliness and dressing
Moving
Breathing
Eating and drinking
Eliminating
Expressing sexuality
Working/playing
Sleeping
Dying

Once the patient's individual problems are highlighted then go on to plan the nursing care and observations needed by the patient and his family.

CHECK LIST

1. ***Professional responsibilities***

e.g. Ward emergencies
Dealing with enquiries
Junior nurses
Confidentiality
Channels of communication
Complaints procedure
The role of Health Visitors/Midwives
The role of Community Health Councils
Awareness of well-known nursing research

2. ***Physiological and Psychological needs***

e.g. Stages of normal physical and mental development
Factors necessary for development to occur
Psychological needs - i.e. Maslow's hierarchy
Effects of hospitalisation and illness on the mental state of the individual
The reaction of individuals to illness

The care of the individual as a patient in conditions related to: (see Master Plan)

3. ***Respiration***

e.g. Respiratory tract investigations
Acute bronchitis
The pneumonias
Respiratory distress
Pulmonary tuberculosis
Asthma
Chronic lung disease
Chest injuries
Pneumothorax
Carcinoma of respiratory tract
Fractured ribs
Childhood respiratory infections
Pleural effusion

4. ***Digestion***

e.g. Alimentary tract investigations
Dysphagia
Oesophageal disorders
Peptic ulcer
Herniae
Appendicitis
Intestinal obstruction
Peritonitis
Diverticulitis
Malabsorption
Ulcerative colitis/ileostomy
Crohn's disease
Malignancy of alimentary tract
Colostomy
Constipation
Jaundice
Gall-bladder disease
Liver diseases
Physiology of portal hypertension

5. ***Excretion***

e.g. Investigations of renal/genito-urinary tract
Causes of haematuria
Reasons for nephrectomy
Infections of kidney
Infections of bladder
Incontinence of urine
Retention of urine
Acute renal failure
Nephrotic syndrome
Chronic renal failure
Prostate gland disorders
Tumours of bladder: benign/malignant
Renal colic/calculi
Water and electrolyte balance

6 *Circulation*

e.g. Investigations of circulatory system
Blood groups, X-matching, transfusion
Anaemia
Haemorrhage
Leukaemia
Angina pectoris
Myocardial infarction
Heart failure
Valve stenosis/incompetence
Subacute bacterial endocarditis
Oedema
Hypertension
Varicose veins/haemorrhoids
Lymphatic disorders
Circulatory deficiency
Blood clotting disorders
Shock

7. *Neurology*

e.g. Epilepsy
Subarachnoid haemorrhage
Cerebrovascular accident
Unconsciousness
Meningitis
Multiple Sclerosis
Pain
Head injury
Types/causes/effects of paralysis
Investigations of neurological disorders
Cataracts
Glaucoma
Corneal abrasions
Blindness
Deafness
Tonsillectomy
Tracheostomy
Laryngectomy
Otitis media

8. ***Hormonal Control***

e.g. Myxoedema
Thyrotoxicosis
Partial thyroidectomy
Diabetes mellitus
Diabetes insipidus
Underactivity of adrenal glands
Overactivity of adrenal glands
Physiological effects of hormones
Cushing's syndrome
Investigation of endocrine dysfunction

9. ***Locomotion***

e.g. Rheumatoid arthritis
Osteoarthritis
Low back pain
Limb amputation
Fractures:
- Potts
- Colles
- Neck of femur
- Shaft of femur
- Tibia/fibula
- Pelvis
- Ribs

Bone healing

10. ***Reproduction***

e.g. Menstruation and menstrual disorders
Infertility
Ectopic pregnancy
Outline normal pregnancy/delivery
Abortion
Uterine fibroids
- prolapse
- malignancy

Venereal diseases
Breast disorders

11. ***Immune response***

e.g. Immunity/immunisation
Autoimmune disorders
Allergies/Anaphylaxis
Communicable diseases: Measles
German Measles
Poliomyelitis
Tetanus
Chickenpox
Mumps

12. ***The Skin***

Burns
e.g. Scalds
Eczema
Psoriasis
Scabies
Fungal infections
Herpes
Wound healing
Pressure sores
Pilonidal sinus

13. ***Drugs and Therapeutic Hazards***

e.g. Legislative control
Infusions
Transfusions
Steroids
Antibiotics
Anticoagulants
Analgesics
Miotics
Mydriatics
Diuretics
Insulin

Case Studies relating to sections 1, 2, 11 and 13 above have not been included but individual questions covering each will be found as part of other case studies. For example questions 45 and 48 refer to drugs and therapeutic hazards although the case study topic is Leukaemia.

RESPIRATION

On each of the following pages you will find a case study followed by 4 related questions. Answers are overleaf.

Tony, aged 16 years, has just left school and has suddenly developed severe bronchospasm. He has been admitted to your ward and the doctor has diagnosed an acute asthmatic attack.

1. Why should you sit Tony in the orthopnoeic position? To

A enable him to use his accessory muscles of respiration
B make room for expansion of the posterior surface of the lungs
C allow for contraction and relaxation of the intercostal muscles
D allow for contraction and relaxation of the diaphragm

2. The *most* dangerous manifestation of an acute asthmatic attack is

A spasm of the muscle of the bronchi
B congestion of the mucous membrane of the main bronchus
C the formation of mucus plugs in the bronchial tree
D the extreme anxiety induced by bronchospasm

3. The cyanosis which occurs during an acute asthmatic attack is due to

A hypoxaemia
B apnoea
C cerebral anoxia
D hyperventilation

4. The primary action of an Intal (Sodium cromoglycate) Spinhaler is to

A dilate the bronchi
B reduce the congestion in the bronchi
C inhibit the allergic response
D control excessive coughing

Answers overleaf

1. A 80%

During an acute asthmatic attack the patient uses the accessory muscles of respiration in an effort to inhale more air. Sitting the patient upright at the beginning of the attack and then allowing him to lean forward onto a bedtable, enables the patient to use the accessory muscles more effectively. Although B, C and D are all correct statements, the question asked for the ***reason*** for the action, therefore A is the correct response.

2. C 60%

The formation of mucus plugs will totally obstruct the flow of air in the already constricted air passages. A, B and D may all occur during an asthmatic attack, however, none of these singly will totally obstruct the air flow and therefore, will not be as serious as C.

3. A 71%

During an acute attack of asthma the alveoli distend in a similar way to emphysema. Insufficient oxygen passes through the alveolar membrane into the bloodstream - this is termed hypoxaemia. Apnoea is cessation of respiration due to temporary reduction of carbon dioxide. Cerebral anoxia is lack of sufficient oxygen to the brain, whilst hyperventilation is over-breathing.

4. C 55%

Sodium Cromoglycate (Intal) acts by inhibiting the allergic reaction in the asthmatic patient which usually follows exposure to specific allergens. By doing this it prevents the results of such an allergy, e.g. bronchospasm, oedema and histamine release, and thus has a primarily prophylactic action. Intal does not directly dilate the bronchi and has no effect on the congestion or coughing.

For the second time in under a year Mr Thomas Jones, aged 76 years, a retired miner who is deaf, is admitted to hospital with an acute exacerbation of chronic bronchitis.

5. **For which of the following reasons does emphysema develop in association with chronic bronchitis:**

   A chronic coughing produces distension and thinning of the alveoli
   B the alveoli dilate due to blockage of the bronchioles by plugs of mucus
   C erosion of the walls of the alveoli occurs due to air pollution
   D paralysis of the muscles takes place in the walls of the alveoli

6. **What is difficulty in breathing whilst lying down called:**

   A apnoea
   B orthopnoea
   C stertorous breathing
   D hyperpnoea

7. **An important principle of management of Mr Jones is the maintenance of**

   A a suitable position
   B cardiac output
   C pulmonary circulation
   D pulmonary ventilation

8. **It is important to give a low concentration of oxygen to a patient with chronic bronchitis because**

   A his hypoxia is the stimulus to the respiratory centre
   B he has an increased sensitivity to carbon dioxide
   C his carbon dioxide levels are raised
   D he may become oxygen dependent

Answers overleaf

5. **B** 66%

If the bronchioles become blocked by mucus, air becomes trapped in the alveoli instead of being exhaled, therefore they become overdistended and loss of elasticity leads to emphysema.

6. **B** 77%

Orthopnoea means difficulty in breathing when lying down.
Apnoea is cessation of breathing. Stertorous breathing is deep, noisy, 'snoring' respirations whilst hyperpnoea is overbreathing.

7. **D** 45%

Pulmonary ventilation means maintenance of an adequate exchange of gases in the lungs not only by a suitable upright position but by other means, e.g. physiotherapy and drugs, and is therefore an important principle of management.

8. **A** 73%

His hypoxia is the stimulus to the respiratory centre. Normally any fall in blood oxygen or increase in carbon dioxide will stimulate the respiratory centre in the medulla and increase breathing rate.
In chronic bronchitis the blood oxygen levels are always lower than normal and the respiratory centre accepts these low levels as 'normal' for the patient. If you then increase blood levels by giving a high percentage of oxygen, this will depress the respiratory centre and reduce breathing rate.

John, a 25 year old student, is admitted to your ward with a spontaneous pneumothorax. He is rather breathless and anxious. The doctor arranges to insert an underwater seal drain.

9. Why will John be breathless? Because

A there will be pressure on the lung
B part of the lung has collapsed
C he is in a shocked condition
D fluid will be accumulating in the pleural cavity

10. Which is the *most* important principle in the management of underwater seal drainage:

A to keep the bottle at a lower level than John's chest
B not to clamp the tubes unnecessarily
C to measure the amount of fluid in the bottle
D to observe that the meniscus is swinging on respiration

11. Before removing the chest drain the doctor will first of all

A order the tube to be clamped for lengthening periods
B order the tube to be clamped for several hours
C ensure the meniscus has stopped swinging as John breathes
D ensure the water is no longer bubbling when John coughs

12. Which of the following is John asked to do immediately before the tube is removed:

A breathe in deeply and breathe out slowly
B breathe out deeply and breathe in slowly
C breathe in deeply and hold his breath
D breathe out deeply and hold his breath

Answers overleaf

9. B 69%

A pneumothorax is air collecting in the pleural space. In spontaneous pneumothorax a small tear in the visceral pleura allows air to enter the pleural space from the lung, causing the lung to collapse. As the mediastinum separates the two sides of the chest, only one lung will be put out of action; breathing is still possible using the other lung, but will be hampered by the mediastinal shift which occurs.

10. A 71%

The aims of an underwater seal are: 1) to allow air and drainage to escape from the pleural cavity, and 2) to prevent any more air or fluid entering. If the bottle is lifted above the level of the chest, fluid would pass from the bottle up the tube and into the pleural cavity.

11. B 21%

After the lungs have fully expanded (as shown by chest X-ray) it is usual to clamp the tube before removal to ensure that the patient does not suffer from pain or undue discomfort. It is normal for the water to bubble when the patient coughs as the air is forced down the drainage tube and into the fluid in the bottle.

12. C 48%

This is to ensure that the lung is fully inflated. Thus when the tube is removed no air can be sucked into the pleural cavity by the patient inhaling. Following the withdrawal of the tube the occluding suture is drawn up and tied or the wound is closed by applying a firm pad of vasoline gauze - again to prevent air entering the pleural cavity.

Mrs Singh is admitted to a side room on the chest ward with a provisional diagnosis of pulmonary tuberculosis. She has a history of recent weight loss, a dry cough and night sweats. Her husband accompanied her as she can speak very little English

13. Why may the doctor ask for an early morning gastric aspiration to be carried out on Mrs Singh? To

A identify the tubercle bacillus
B test acidity of gastric juice
C test for tuberculous peritonitis
D discover the reason for weight loss

14. Why was Mrs Singh initially prescribed a combination of three drugs:

A to lessen the side effects of any one drug
B in case she has the infection elsewhere
C because the tubercle bacillus may be resistant to one or two drugs
D so that she will not have to have daily injections

15. When will the result be received of a sputum specimen sent for culture of tubercle bacillus to the bacteriology department:

A within 24 hours
B in 2-4 days
C after 1 week
D 6-8 weeks later

16. After she has commenced her treatment, Mrs Singh complains of vertigo. The *most* likely cause is

A Rifamcin
B Streptomycin
C Isoniazid
D Ethambutol

Answers overleaf

13. A 24%

Tuberculous patients sometimes have difficulty in coughing up sputum and tend to swallow it. As the tubercle bacillus has a protective layer it is not destroyed by the hydrochloric acid in the stomach and can therefore be identified.

14. C 76%

Three drugs are always given at the beginning of treatment otherwise resistance to the drugs occurs. If the treatment is started with two drugs about half the patients are resistant to the action of one drug after about 3 months. Given in combination the development of resistance is minimal. Once sensitivities of the organism is known, treatment can be continued with a combination of two sensitive drugs. (Drugs must be given for at least 9 months.)

15. D 22%

It takes 6 to 8 weeks for culture as the tubercle bacillus is slow growing, only dividing approximately once in every 24 hours.

16. B 56%

In large doses Streptomycin may damage the auditory (8th cranial) nerve. Signs of auditory damage include high pitched tinnitus and vertigo.
Side effects of the other drugs:-
Rifamcin - due to its solubility in water it may cause reddish discolouration of urine, sputum and sweat.
Ethambutol - is toxic to the optic nerve and vision should be tested at regular intervals.
Isoniazid - may neutralise vitamin B6 present in the body with resultant possibility of peripheral neuropathy. Prophylactic pyridoxin (vitamin B6) if given with the drugs prevents this from occurring.

Mrs Kaur, a widow who has 2 small children aged 4 and 6 years, has a history of weight loss, coughing and night sweats.
A provisional diagnosis of pulmonary tuberculosis has been made.

17. Which of the following drugs would damage the eighth cranial nerve

A Streptomycin
B Isoniazid
C Para-amino Salicylic acid
D Ethambutol

18. Which of the following laboratory tests is most likely to identify the tubercle bacillus in Mrs Kaur's sputum:

A culture and sensitivity
B acid fast bacilli
C cytology and cells
D surfactant estimation

19. Which of the following is the *most* common complication of haemorrhage in the tuberculous patient:

A spread of tuberculosis to other parts of the lung
B hypovolaemic shock
C distension of the alveoli
D hyperchromic anaemia

20. Which of the following would be used specifically in the treatment of pulmonary tuberculosis:

A Isoniazid
B BCG Vaccination
C Salicylic Acid
D Pyridoxine

Answers overleaf

17. A 42%

Streptomycin damages the eighth cranial nerve. Isoniazid passes through the meninges and is a useful drug in tuberculous meningitis. Para-amino salicylic acid has direct action on the tubercle bacillus and delays streptomycin resistance. Side effects include nausea, vomiting, diarrhoea, rashes, liver damage.
Ethambutol is an anti-tuberculous drug. It occasionally produces inflammation of the optic nerve and this usually resolves when the drug is discontinued.

18. B 38%

The tubercle bacillus is acid and alcohol fast. (After the bacillus has been stained the colour is not removed by either acid or alcohol.) Culture and sensitivity ***may*** be carried out but mycobacterium tuberculosis are not always identifiable by this method.
Surfactant is secreted by the alveolar membrane.

19. A 19%

A lesion which is adherent to a vein erodes its walls and pours bacilli into the blood. If the vein is a systemic vein then dissemination of tuberculosis to other parts of the lungs occurs.
Haemorrhage is not sufficiently profuse to produce hypovolaemic shock. Inflammation of the alveoli accous rather than distension. D is a manifestation of pernicious anaemia.

20. A 52%

Bacille Calmette-Guerin (B.C.G.) when injected into humans causes only local lesions, but stimulates the development of immunity effective against tuberculosis. It is not used for treatment of tuberculosis. Salicylic acid is used in the treatment of some skin diseases i.e. plantar warts.
Sodium aminosalicylate is used in the treatment of tuberculosis when first-line drugs cause unacceptable side effects or the organism is resistant to treatment.
Pyridoxine, one of the vitamin B group, would not be used specifically in the treatment of tuberculosis.

CIRCULATION

Mr Alcock is a 65 year old retired fitter. He lives alone having lost his wife 3 months previously and has been admitted in congestive cardiac failure. He has been very ill for 2 days at home and has broken skin over his sacrum.

21. Which of the following groups of signs and symptoms are *most* likely:

    A gravitational oedema, hypertension and bradycardia
    B pulmonary oedema, dyspnoea and polyuria
    C distended neck veins, cyanosis and tachycardia
    D chest pain, cold extremities and stertorous breathing

22. Which of the following drugs would be ordered intravenously by the doctor for immediate administration:

    A Aminophylline and Frusemide
    B Digoxin and Salbutamol
    C Practolol and Lignocaine
    D Pethidine and Diazepam

23. Which of the following is the reason why Mr Alcock was ordered oxygen at 24% concentration. To

    A commence oxygen therapy gradually and slowly increase concentration
    B prevent excess carbon dioxide accumulating in the blood
    C stimulate the respiratory centre to speed up respiratory rate
    D maintain the present situation with regard to respiratory stimulus

24. Which of the following nursing objectives would be *most* reasonable regarding the broken area on his sacrum. To

    A heal the area in 2 days
    B prevent infection and relieve pressure
    C apply a non-adhesive sterile dressing
    D review the area 2 hourly

Answers overleaf

21. C 52%

This patient is in congestive cardiac failure therefore the veins are distended due to generalised venous congestion. There is cyanosis due to poor gaseous exchange because of his chest condition and a failing circulation preventing good tissue oxygenation. Tachycardia occurs because the failing heart beats more rapidly and less effectively.

22. A 81%

Aminophylline is a bronchodilator and therefore would be required in order to aid oxygenation. Frusemide is a diuretic and as this patient is oedematous the drug would be required.
B - neither of these drugs are often given intravenously.
C and D are unlikely.

23. D 35%

As a sufferer of chronic bronchitis, Mr Alcock has been breathing as a result of oxygen lack for many years. If his oxygen concentration is high then his stimulus to breathe would be disturbed. In order to maintain the present situation he is given a 24% concentration of oxygen so that stimulation of the respiratory centre is maintained.

24. B 72%

A nursing objective is an attainable goal that is reasonable and can be evaluated in a set space of time. A is too ambitious; C and D are both practices which should be included in the nursing care plan and are not objectives; B therefore is the correct answer.

Mrs Parry, aged 60, is admitted to your ward as an emergency. She awoke suddenly during the night with an attack of severe breathlessness. She has been diagnosed as having left ventricular failure and has been admitted for treatment and investigations.

25. Which of the following is the commonest cause of left ventricular failure:

A hypertension
B chronic bronchitis
C coronary artery disease
D rheumatic heart disease

26. Where does oedema occur initially in left ventricular failure:

A sacrum
B ankles
C lungs
D legs

27. You are asked to administer 250 micrograms of Digoxin. You have a solution containing 0.5 milligrams per millilitre of Digoxin. You should give

A 2 mls
B 0.5 mls
C 5 mls
D 0.05 mls

28. Which of the following is a symptom of potassium depletion:

A vomiting
B cramp
C muscle weakness
D hypotension

Answers overleaf

25. A 42%

In order to pump blood into the aorta against the increased resistance the left ventricle hypertrophies. Eventually the left ventricle may no longer be able to do this and so left ventricular failure occurs. Chronic bronchitis usually causes right sided heart failure initially. Coronary artery disease and valvular disease may cause left ventricular failure but neither are the commonest.

26. C 56%

In left ventricular failure the weakened left ventricle of the heart does not effectively pump blood into the aorta. This causes blood to build up in the left atrium and pulmonary vessels. Pressure within the pulmonary vessels rises so that it causes pulmonary oedema, forcing fluid into the lung tissue.

27. B 46%

One millilitre contains 0.5 milligrams (500 micrograms)

250 micrograms = 0.25 milligrams, therefore:-

A) 2 mls of this solution would give 1 mg of Digoxin.
2 x 0.5 mgs = 1 mg

B) 0.5 mls/½/ ml would give 0.25 mgs or 250 micrograms.
1 ml = 0.5 mgs
½ ml = 0.25 mgs

C) 5 mls of this solution would give 2.5 mgs.
5 x 0.5 mgs 2.5 mgs

D) 0.05 mls of this solution would give 0.025 mgs.
1 ml = 0.5 mgs
0.5 ml = 0.25 mgs
0.05 ml = 0.025 mg

28. C 34%

Muscle weakness occurs due to loss of potassium, it is essential for effective nerve conduction and hence the response of muscles to stimuli. Thiazide diuretics may cause anorexia, nausea, vomiting. Depletion of calcium caused by diuretics may cause muscle cramp. Hypotension is not a symptom of potassium loss, although Thiazide diuretics have some lowering effect on the blood pressure.

Four days after surgery Mr Black complains of left calf pain. The doctor diagnoses a deep vein thrombosis and prescribes anticoagulant therapy.

29. Which of the following nursing plans might have *best* prevented the occurrence of his complication:

A pre-operative anticoagulant therapy and urinalysis
B constant supervision in the post-operative period
C explanation of the need for movement reinforced by encouragement
D passive leg exercise performed 2 hourly by the nurse

30. Which of the following statements about anticoagulant therapy is correct:

A heparin, if used for more than 48 hours results in reactionary thrombosis
B oral anticoagulants interfere with vitamin K synthesis
C the antidote to warfarin is protamine sulphate
D heparin dissolves thrombin in the bloodstream

31. Which of the following care plans is now appropriate:

A regular urinalysis, observations of respirations, and noting the presence of any chest pain
B observation of stools, strict bed rest and positioning of pillow under the legs
C use of a bed cradle, calf circumference measurements and fluid balance
D monitoring pain in leg and observing for ankle oedema, cardiac arrhythmias and cough

32. Thrombosis may occur following surgery because of

A increased viscosity of blood due to pre-operative starving and anaemia due to blood loss
B damage to vein wall due to handling in theatre and anaesthetic drugs
C use of atropine pre-operatively and increase in serum prothrombin level
D paralysis of muscle in groups and increase in platelet stickiness

Answers overleaf

29. C 78%

Had Mr Black been told specifically why he needed to move after operation and this had been reinforced by the nurses then the risk of deep vein thrombosis would have been reduced.
(See "Information, Prescription against pain" R.C.N. Publications, Author J. Hayward)

30. B 35%

Vitamin K is required for the production of prothrombin in the liver. The oral anti-coagulants e.g. warfarin, interfere with this synthesis of vitamin K and therefore the level of prothrombin in the blood is reduced. A is an incorrect statement. The antidote to warfarin is vitamin K. Protamine sulphate is the antidote to heparin. The action of heparin is to prevent further clotting in the blood stream.

31. A 38%

The further adjustments to Mr Black's care plan are aimed at detecting any side effects of the drugs that he has now been prescribed and also to observe for the complications of pulmonary embolism which may be the result of the deep vein thrombosis. The regular urinalysis will show up haematuria and the observation of respiration and colour for chest pain will highlight the possibility of pulmonary embolism. Positioning a pillow under the legs would be a dangerous practice as it constricts venous return. In C a bed cradle would be useful and some doctors do like regular calf circumference measurements but a fluid balance record if this is not already being carried out will not be of particular use. D - monitoring pain in the leg and observing for ankle oedema are both quite reasonable things for the nurse to do but there isn't really any reason why she should specifically look for cardiac arrhythmias.

32. D 14%

The muscle groups are paralysed during general anaesthesia and operation and consequently venous return is somewhat inhibited. There is also an increase in platelet stickiness following anaesthetic and operation, although the reasons for this are not particularly clear.

John, aged 4 years, is a known haemophiliac. He is admitted to your ward with a haemarthrosis of his left knee.

33. Which group of observations would be most appropriate for the nurse to carry out:

A ½ hourly pulse and 4 hourly blood pressure
B hourly measurement of the knee and ½ hourly pulse
C temperature 4 hourly and measurement of the knee daily
D blood pressure and temperature hourly until stable

34. Which drugs are likely to be prescribed for John:

A Episkapron and Nepenthe
B Cryoprecipitate and antibiotics
C Nepenthe and Cryoprecipitate
D antibiotics and Episkapron

35. The amount of drugs given to control the bleed is based upon the patient's

A platelet count
B age
C factor VIII
D weight

36. Which of the following will John require:

A passive movements to his knee joint as soon as the pain decreases
B immobilisation of the knee joint until the bleeding ceases
C immobilisation of the knee joint for a minimum of 2 weeks
D active movements of the knee joint to prevent deformity

Answers overleaf

33. B 62%

The knee circumference and pulse will indicate the severity of bleeding. The blood pressure is unlikely to fall, and it is the extent of the bleed into the joint which is important. Temperature recordings are not significant.

34. C 19%

Cryoprecipitate contains factor VIII and Nepenthe will relieve the pain. Any bleed into a joint is acutely painful and results in swelling because of the restricted space.

35. C 41%

There are varying degrees of haemophilia. Those children with a very low level of factor VIII need to have their levels raised in order to control the bleed.

36. B 63%

It is important to immobilise the joint until bleeding has ceased but it should not be immobilised for any longer than is necessary. Passive movements may begin as soon as bleeding stops.

William Jackson, a 42 year old self-employed plumber, is admitted to hospital with a myocardial infarction. He is suffering from chest pain and this is relieved by Diamorphine, but he appears extremely anxious on admission to the ward.

37. What does the term myocardial infarction mean:

A blockage of the coronary artery
B arteriosclerotic changes in cardiac muscle
C artherosclerotic changes in cardiac muscle
D death of cardiac muscle

38. When attaching Mr Jackson to a cardiac monitor the priority of the nurse is to:

A establish good skin/electrode contact
B explain why the procedure is necessary
C shave his chest prior to the application of electrodes
D explain that Mr Jackson must lie still

39. Which of the following is vital whilst taking Mr Jackson's nursing history. The nurse should

A establish his pattern of daily living
B complete the nursing history form fully
C seek information from his medical records
D discuss with him his perception of the situation

40. When assessing Mr Jackson's nursing needs it is of *prime* importance to

A administer sedatives as prescribed
B encourage Mr Jackson to rest
C allow Mr Jackson to talk freely and listen
D record pulse and apex beat 2 hourly

Answers overleaf

37. D 80%

Myocardial infarction means death of cardiac muscle although a blockage of the coronary artery will cause the infarction. Arterio or atherosclerotic changes in the coronary arteries are predisposing factors which may contribute towards development of a coronary thrombosis.

38. B 57%

You should have noted from the history that Mr Jackson is extremely anxious, therefore the priority is to explain why the procedure is necessary. This will help to reduce his anxiety and by lowering his anxiety level you are minimising the physiological effects of stress, i.e. tachycardia, vasoconstriction, thus reducing the strain on his already strained heart.

39. D 45%

The purpose of a nursing history is to devise an individual plan of care based on information received, so the patient's perception of the situation is vital in planning realistic nursing care. Although A, B and C may be carried out, none are vital but A is also important. When planning care the patients abilities and wishes must be considered - hence D is *vital*.

40. C 24%

Allow Mr Jackson to express his fear and worries to reduce anxiety and stress which may delay recovery. Additionally, only C is directly concerned with assessment of the patient's needs, the other distractors are all aspects of giving or planning care.

Simon aged 4 years, is to be admitted to your ward with suspected leukaemia. He is an only child and is accompanied by his unmarried mother.

41. Which of the following is the commonest type of leukaemia in children:

A acute myeloid
B chronic myeloid
C acute lymphoblastic
D chronic lymphoblastic

42. What are the symptoms of anaemia and purpura likely to be due to:

A leukaemic infiltration of the liver and spleen
B decrease in the manufacture of all blood cells
C crowding out of the marrow by immature white cells
D alteration in the permeability of the capillary wall

43. Which of the following are the most likely investigations:

A bone marrow puncture and E.M.I. scan
B lumbar puncture and bone marrow puncture
C peripheral blood picture and E.M.I. scan
D lumbar puncture and gland biopsy

44. Which of the following aspects of nursing management must be included in the care plan:

A monitoring of his temperature and good fluid intake
B high protein diet and free visiting
C play therapy and vitamin C supplements
D quiet environment and diet containing extra iron

Answers overleaf

41. C 44%

85% of leukaemia in childhood is acute lymphoblastic. The remaining 15% is usually acute myeloid.

42. C 46%

The increase in immature lymphocytes leads to a decrease of erythrocytes, neutrophils and thrombocytes from crowding out in the marrow. A is therefore incorrect; B is wrong - there is an increase in the manufacture of lymphocytes; D is wrong - there is no alteration in the permeability of the capillary wall.

43. B 35%

Bone marrow puncture will demonstrate the lymphoblasts. The lumbar puncture will determine whether there is a central nervous system, involvement, blast cells can be seen in the C.S.F. A and C are incorrect, an E.M.I. scan will not help. D - a gland biopsy is unnecessary.

44. A 26%

Simon is very prone to infection as his neutrophil count is decreased, his lymphocytes are immature. A good fluid intake is important to keep his mouth clean - he is unlikely to be eating well.
High protein diet is inappropriate at this stage, there should be restriction on visitors with infections.
Vitamin C supplements will not help - he can have fruit juices which he will enjoy more. Although he is anaemic he may not be iron deficient. He should not necessarily need to be quiet; children enjoy company and activity going on around them even if they are unable to participate.

Julie is a 7 year old only child. On admission to a children's ward, it has been necessary to nurse Julie in a side room as her diagnosis is acute lymphocytic leukaemia. She will be treated using cytotoxic drugs by combination therapy.

45. Which one of the following is a common toxic effect of Cyclophosphamide:

A tinnitus
B diarrhoea
C polycythaemia
D alopecia

46. Which of the following methods would most effectively protect Julie from infection:

A all persons entering her room should wear masks and gowns
B visitors should be limited to her immediate family
C large doses of various antibiotics should be given
D her diet should contain adequate vitamin C

47. The thrombocytopenia associated with Julie's condition would probably result in

A body temperature of 40° C
B increased tendency to paraesthesia
C bleeding of gums
D increasing fatigue and pallor

48. During administration of a blood transfusion Julie complains of loin pain. The nurse should

A observe her condition, particularly the temperature
B stop the transfusion and notify the doctor
C measure the urinary output and record the amount
D assess the transfusion site for extravasation

Answers overleaf

45. D 55%

A noise in the ears such as ringing, buzzing or roaring, (tinnitus) is not a common toxic effect caused by Cyclophosphamide, nor even an unexpected side effect. Upsets of the gastro-intestinal tract often occur following treatment but usually result in nausea and vomiting which may be reduced by the prior administration of an anti-emetic drug. An increase in the total red blood cell mass (polycythaemia) would be most unlikely as the drug is more likely to produce a depression of bone marrow function resulting in reduced formation of erythrocytes, granulocytes and platelets.

46. A 61%

Restriction of visitors would not effectively protect Julie from infection unless the additional wearing of masks and gowns was adopted. Large doses of antibiotics may have some effect in protecting the patient but would not be very effective without some form of 'reverse barrier nursing'. A diet containing adequate vitamin C would not be the ***most*** effective protection of Julie. Supplementary vitamins may be given in addition to diet to endeavour to improve the patient's state of health which indirectly may offer some protection.

47. C 38%

Pyrexia associated with the patient's condition may be as a result of infection. Thrombocytopenia is a decrease in the number of platelets in the blood and is likely to make the patient more prone to bleeding especially of the gums. An abnormal sensation such as burning or prickling, often described as 'pins and needles' (paraesthesia) may accompany treatment with cytotoxic drugs such as Cyclophosphamide and is a side-effect of treatment but it is not produced as an effect of a decrease in the number of platelets. Julie's condition may feature increasing fatigue and pallor which may be a result of depression of the bone marrow causing anaemia.

48. B 59%

The most important action the nurse should take would be to stop the transfusion and notify the doctor. The other answers would be associated with nursing any patient who was having a blood transfusion. (Extravasation is redness and oedema around the site.)

Mrs Brown is a 60 year old housewife who suffers from congestive heart failure, she lives with her husband in a large council house. She is an obese woman and gets breathless easily on exertion, she also has oedema of her feet and ankles which makes it difficult to wear shoes. Mrs Brown's condition has deteriorated during the last few months often waking her during the night, so she has been admitted to hospital for relief of her symptoms.

49. A relatively *uncommon* feature of congestive heart failure is

A cough
B scanty urinary output
C severe cardiac pain
D breathlessness

50. Mrs Brown's oedema is most likely to be due to

A raised arterial pressure
B raised venous pressure
C lowered arterial pressure
D lowered venous pressure

51. The purpose of nursing Mrs Brown in the upright position is to

A encourage the movement of fluid from the heart and lungs
B increase the arterial blood pressure
C assist cardiac emptying by compressing the heart
D make breathing easier

52. Paroxysmal nocturnal dyspnoea is primarily due to

A accumulation of serous fluid in alveolar spaces
B obstruction of bronchi by mucoid secretions
C compression of lung tissue by a dilated heart
D restriction of respiratory movement by ascites

Answers overleaf

49. C 60%

Pulmonary oedema and reduced blood flow to the kidneys because of lowered cardiac output account for the cough, oliguria and dyspnoea of congestive cardiac failure.
Severe cardiac pain is an uncommon feature.

50. B 63%

The congestion in the lungs and venous system causes a rise in venous pressure. This prevents reabsorption of tissue fluid, thus causing oedema as the venous pressure is greater than the osmotic pressure in the capillary.

51. D 74%

By nursing Mrs Brown in the upright position pressure on the diaphragm by abdominal organs will be reduced, thereby facilitating greater contraction. As a result, the volume within the thoracic cavity is increased and lung expansion similarly increased.

52. A 54%

Excessive pulmonary fluid in the alveolar spaces impairs oxygen diffusion into the capillaries and cyanosis increases. Whilst asleep Mrs Brown will tend to slip down the bed into a supine position which will place an added strain on her already laboured breathing. Thus she is likely to wake up at night gasping for breath as a result of her cardiac failure - hence the term "cardiac asthma" or paroxysmal (spasmodic) nocturnal (at night) dyspnoea (breathlessness).

Mrs Joan Smith. aged 38 years, is recovering from having had a total abdominal hysterectomy three days ago. On admission she weighed 59 kilograms and had been smoking 20 cigarettes a day. Her recovery so far has been satisfactory but today she has a slight rise in temperature and whilst you are attending to her, complains that one of her legs is aching. You suspect a deep vein thrombosis.

53. **Which of the following would be the *most* likely sign or symptom:**

    A on examination her whole leg will be quite swollen
    B the pain will be worse on walking
    C Kernig's sign will be positive
    D there will be an area of redness

54. **Which of the following will be the *main* predisposing factor in the development of Mrs Smith's deep vein thrombosis? Her:**

    A weight
    B smoking
    C age
    D operation site

55. **Which of the following observations is *most* important after the diagnosis of deep vein thrombosis has been made:**

    A sputum
    B temperature
    C pulse
    D blood pressure

56. **When Mrs Smith is discharged home on anticoagulants she will be advised to:**

    A test her urine for blood
    B report any vomiting immediately
    C not take aspirin
    D get out of bed slowly in the morning

Answers overleaf

53. B 59%

Options A and may subsequently arise as a result of a deep vein thrombosis (phlebothrombosis) but pain which increases in severity when the patient walks is most likely because of the increased muscle pressure on the area and spasm of vessels affected.

54. B 62%

59 kgs (about 10 stones) may not be excessively heavy although the question does not state Mrs Smith's height in relation to weight. Her age and operation site will not contribute to the formation of a deep vein thrombosis but smoking will, for one of the effects of smoking is to constrict blood vessels. This then is the main predisposing factor although A could also play some part.

55. A 71%

A potential hazard facing Mrs Smith following the development of her deep vein thrombosis is that of pulmonary embolism should the clot dislodge and travel via the inferior vena cava, right atrium and ventricle and pulmonary arteries, to the lung. If the embolism blocks a small vessel the patient will complain of dyspnoea and chest pain and may produce bloodstained sputum as red cells from the vessels of the infarcted area exude into the alveoli.

56. C 73%

Aspirin irritates gastric mucosa and can cause haematemesis. If the patient also was receiving anticoagulant therapy with a resulting prolongation of clotting time then any gastric bleeding would be enhanced and put the patient at severe risk. Haematuria is one of the early signs of anticoagulant overdosage but it would seem more feasible simply to tell Mrs Smith to note the colour of her urine rather than expect her to test it for blood.

EXCRETION

Mr Spanswick, aged 64, a retired mechanic, is re-admitted following discharge 6 weeks ago with a recurrence of nephrotic syndrome. He lives with his wife and daughter who is getting married in two weeks time. On admission his blood pressure is 100/60, temperature 37° C and respirations 20/minute.

57. Which of the following is likely to be highlighted during Mr Spanswick's initial assessment:

A polyuria and loin pain
B albuminuria and oedema
C dysuria and dehydration
D back pain and vomiting

58. Which of the following would be ordered by the doctor for intravenous administration:

A dextrose/saline plus potassium to correct his fluid and electrolyte balance
B plasma protein fraction to replace protein lost in urine
C packed cells to treat anaemia secondary to renal disease
D Manitol to encourage a good diuresis

59. Which of the following goals would be *most* important to Mr Spanswick initially:

A becoming symptom free and off medication
B being able to enjoy a normal diet
C obtaining relief of nocturia and nausea
D attending his daughter's wedding in 2 weeks time

60. Which of the following statements about Mr Spanswick's blood pressure recording is most accurate. It is

A normal and does not warrant action
B low due to diminished blood viscosity
C low due to failure of renin angiotensin mechanism
D normal but should be re-checked

Answers overleaf

57. **B** 78%

In nephrotic syndrome the filtration mechanism in the Bowman's capsule is damaged and albumin, a plasma protein, escapes from the capillary network into the tubule and is subsequently excreted in the urine in large amounts. Plasma albumin levels are therefore lowered which causes the osmotic pressure of the blood to fall and fluid which would normally be reabsorbed is now retained within the tissues. The initial assessment is therefore going to highlight B - albuminuria and oedema. A, C and D are features associated with other renal disorders.

58. **B** 57%

The most important consideration is the replacement of the albumin which is being lost by the mechanism described above. The solution which would most certainly be ordered by the doctor is B.
Dextrose/saline would not help to correct fluid balance as it would not correct the cause of the imbalance i.e. albumin loss.
Anaemia may be present but is much more commonly asociated with chronic renal disease. Manitol would not be a diuretic of choice as correction of the serum albumin levels is essential.

59. **D** 70%

When deciding the answer to this question it is important to note that this is Mr Spanswick's second admission so he will already be familiar with his treatment. Whilst at home, the whole family will have been involved in the wedding preparations then only two weeks before the event he is suddenly re-admitted to hospital. It is very likely that D - attending his daughter's wedding will be uppermost in his mind.
Becoming symptom free will be important but probably of secondary importance in relation to the prospects of attending the wedding. He is likely to be aware that medication will continue long term. Diet will also be a familiar part of his treatment and accepted as a means to recovery. He may not have the problems in C.

60. **B** 26%

Mr Spanswick's blood pressure is 100/60 mmHg. This is not a normal recording for a man of his age, it is far too low. This excludes distractors A and D as both state that it is normal. It has already been ascertained that because of the albuminuria the plasma albumin levels will be low. This will result in low blood volume and low blood viscosity. The correct answer is therefore B. The renin-angiotensin mechanism is unlikely to fail because of nephrotic syndrome.

Angela Morris, a single girl of 18, is admitted to the medical unit with a diagnosis of acute pyelonephritis. She is 4 months pregnant and accompanied by her parents who are extremely anxious.

61. Which of the following are you most likely to discover when assessing Angela on admission. That she

A is sweating, pyrexial and has loin pain
B has oedema, oliguria and lower abdominal pain
C has dysuria, raised blood pressure and oedema
D is hypotensive, pyrexial and has diarrhoea

62. Which of the following approaches to Angela would be best as she is pregnant:

A avoid mentioning it as she has enough to contend with
B try to discover how she feels about it
C address questions to her parents and avoid distressing Angela
D try to discover her attitudes to termination of pregnancy

63. Which of the following amounts of fluid should Angela be given each 24 hours:

A 500 ml plus equivalent of previous day's output
B 1,500 ml
C 3,000 ml
D 5,000 ml less equivalent of previous day's output

64. Which of the following will help determine treatment:

A intravenous urogram
B amount of blood and protein in urine
C results of mid- stream urine test
D anti- streptolysin "O" titre

Answers overleaf

61. A 59%

Sweating and pyrexia are always associated with acute infections and loin pain is a specific characteristic of pyelonephritis due to the inflammation of the renal tissue and kidney pelvis. Oedema is not associated with this condition as the kidneys still maintain fluid balance. Oliguria may be present if Angela is becoming dehydrated due to sweating. The pain is usually loin pain, not lower abdominal. Blood pressure may be slightly raised due to stress but should normalise. Dysuria may well be present.

62. B 74%

Angela may have a lot of anxieties and problems which, as she is single, she may not have discussed with anyone. This would be a good opportunity for her to talk to someone who is not personally involved. Not mentioning the subject could cause her even more distress as she may have no-one to talk to about it. It may be that she wants the baby and is afraid her condition could harm it. Her parents may not even know that she is pregnant and therefore C would breach confidentiality. It must not be assumed that Angela wants a termination and at four months this would be difficult.

63. C 21%

3,000 ml is an increase on the normal daily intake and will be required to correct dehydration from sweating and to "flush" the kidneys of infective material.

64. C 40%

Pyelonephritis is an infective condition and treatment is based on recognition of the causative organism and finding an appropriate antibiotic to treat it with. The only means of finding out this information is by doing a mid-stream urine test. An intravenous urogram is an investigation which may be carried out although it will not provide any information regarding the infective agent and treatment cannot be based upon the results. Blood and protein may well be present in the urine and a lessening amount may be an indication of improvement but not relevant as a basis for treatment.

Joanna, aged 17 years, is admitted following a diagnosis of acute nephritis. Joanna is pyrexial and has marked peri-orbital oedema, she seems particularly distressed as her art college examinations are due the following week.

65. Which of the following is the most likely factor related to the development of acute nephritis:

A frequency of micturition
B examination revision stress
C upper respiratory tract infection
D increasing domestic tension

66. Which of the following problems is Joanna's initial nursing assessment likely to highlight:

A headache, raised blood urea, pain in back
B raised blood pressure, vomiting, pain
C oedema, fever, pain in back
D vomiting, sore throat, haematuria

67. When designing a nursing plan, priority should be given to

A early mobilisation, fluid restriction and temperature observation
B bed rest, diet and observation of intake and output
C observation of urine, relief of pain and diet
D position in bed, relief of oedema and fluid restriction

68. Which of the following most aptly describes urine in the early stages of acute nephritis:

A dilute with ketones and casts
B concentrated with albumin and sugar
C contains blood, pus and ketones
D contains casts, albumin and blood

Answers overleaf

65. C 65%

Acute nephritis is often associated with an infective condition caused by the haemolytic streptococci. This micro-organism commonly causes tonsillitis and upper respiratory tract conditions. Toxins produced by the organism cause an allergic reaction in the glomerulus - it is therefore an allergic disorder.

66. C 53%

Oedema is caused by the reduced glomerular filtration and increased reabsorption of water and salts by the tubules. Fever is present because it is associated with acute inflammation in the glomerulus. The back pain is caused by this inflammatory process. Headache is a very non-specific feature which may or may not be present. Raised blood urea and back pain may both be present but the blood urea is linked to medical and not nursing assessment. Pain is not specific enough, the pain is localised and the place should be stated. Blood pressure may well be raised and vomiting could occur but again is rather non-specific. Sore throat is not likely to be present as the acute nephritis usually manifests itself 2 - 3 weeks after the initial infection. Joanna may also have haematuria and vomiting.

67. B 47%

The three main principles of nursing care in acute nephritis are i) maintain rest, ii) control protein and salt intake and iii) maintain fluid balance. Early mobilization is contra-indicated. Observation of the urine is important but not a priority. Position in bed may be best determined by Joanna herself. Relief of oedema is rather vague and is achieved by maintaining fluid balance and dietary control of protein and salt intake.

68. D 54%

This condition does not result in sugar or ketones being present in the urine. After exclusion of the distractors containing these two things the answer must be D. Albumin, casts and blood appear in the urine because of the inflammation in the glomerulus - the spaces in the Bowman's capsule enlarge and larger molecules than usual are allowed to filter into the tubule.

Carol Williams, aged 30 years, who is due to be married later this year, is found to be suffering from chronic renal failure.

69. Which of the following is *most* hazardous. An elevated

A serum calcium
B serum albumin
C serum bicarbonate
D serum potassium

70. Which of the following are likely to be present during the early course of the disease:

A raised urine output, raised specific gravity
B raised urine output, lowered specific gravity
C lowered urine output, lowered specific gravity
D lowered urine output, raised specific gravity

71. What does the term renal threshold indicate. The

A amount of urine produced
B ability to excrete sodium
C amount of substance reabsorbed
D ability to concentrate urine

72. Following insertion of an arterio-venous shunt the nurse should call the doctor quickly if she observes

A oliguria
B non-pulsating shunt
C hypertension
D inflammation of the shunt site

Answers overleaf

69. D 40%

In chronic renal failure there are many disturbances of electrolytes and changes of blood chemistry especially raised levels of urea, creatinine, sodium and potassium. Each is damaging to the patient but hyperkalaemia (raised potassium levels) may cause a cardiac arrest and is therefore the ***most*** hazardous of those listed.

70. B 13%

As the nephrons become damaged they are unable to concentrate the urine by reabsorbing water, therefore urinary output will be increased with a reduced concentration of waste products. When the majority of nephrons are damaged urinary output generally diminishes although this is in the more advanced stage of renal failure, commonly termed "end stage renal failure".

71. C 55%

The amount of a substance reabsorbed denotes the renal threshold. For glucose it is 10 mmols/litre of blood. If the blood glucose level is above this there is an increased amount in the filtrate and the cells of the proximal convoluted tubule are unable to reabsorb it all. Therefore some glucose is excreted in the urine.

72. B 50%

Following insertion of an arterio- venous shunt for haemodialysis you should ensure the shunt is pulsating. The shunt may clot easily thus delaying access to the bloodstream for dialysis and the nurses role is to detect any change in the pulsation of the shunt so that clotting can be prevented or treated quickly once it has arisen.

Mrs Johnson, aged 35 years, is to have a partial thyroidectomy in two weeks time. She has been having conservative treatment with Carbimazole for the past eighteen months, and the relief of symptoms is now greatly reduced.

73. Which of the following drugs will be prescribed pre-operatively:

A Neo-Mercazole
B potassium iodide
C thyroxine sodium
D liothyronine sodium

74. Which of the following is most important pre-operatively. To

A nurse Mrs Johnson in a quiet part of the ward
B explain fully the nature and purpose of surgery
C administer prescribed medications on time
D ensure that nurses are aware of possibly complications of thyroid surgery

75. Three days pre-operatively Mrs Johnson complains of a mild cough with no other obvious symptoms. This is *most* likely to be due to

A a respiratory infection
B the side effect of gastritis from the drug
C her toxic goitre obstructing the trachea
D bronchial secretions stimulated by the prescribed drug

76. Which of the following changes in the gland is a specific aim of pre-operative medication. That it be

A greatly reduced in size
B firmer and avascular
C softer and less vascular
D firmer and less vascular

Answers overleaf

73. B 60%

Potassium iodide controls the output of thyroxine from the gland and reduces the glands vascularity which is an important factor when reducing the risks of the post-operative complication haemorrhage. Neo-Mercazole has minimal effects upon vascularity but is used prior to potassium iodide to reduce/inhibit thyroid function only.
Thyroxine sodium is used in myxoedema or cretinism to replace deficiency of the hormone. Liothyronine sodium is used to aid diagnosis and again has no effect upon the gland which would aid surgery.

74. C 80%

It is important to explain fully the nature and purpose of the operation to Mrs Johnson and also to nurse her in a quiet part of the ward as she is likely to be agitated as a result of her thyrotoxicosis.
However, the ***most*** important aspect of care is to ensure that all drugs, including the premedication, are given on time.

75. D 57%

Potassium is also a mild expectorant, therefore the new symptom of cough is not unusual when the medicine is given for thyroid surgery preparation. The other symptoms do not relate to the medication.

76. D 62%

Potassium iodide is given to reduce vascularity and to firm the glandular tissue which aids the surgeon. The three distractors would not help surgery as a firm tissue is easier to both hold and incise especially when the likelihood to bleed is also reduced.

Alan is 8 years old and is admitted to your ward in a hyperglycaemic coma. His mother accompanies him. She is very distressed as he was not known to be a diabetic.

77. Which of the following groups of clinical features are likely to be present:

A tachycardia, low blood pressure and clammy skin
B high blood pressure, bradycardia and Kussmaul respirations
C dehydration, tachycardia and low blood pressure
D glycosuria, bradycardia and dehydration

78. Which of the following is Alan's history most likely to include? Recent

A thirst, increased appetite and enuresis
B weight gain, polyuria and giddy attacks
C pruritus, anorexia and thirst
D polyuria, thirst and diarrhoca

79. Which of the following will form part of Alan's future management:

A teach Alan to give his own injections
B teach his mother to give his injections
C teach Alan and his mother to give his injections
D arrange for the district nurse to give his injections

80. Which of the following is responsible for the induction of the coma in hyperglycaemia:

A hyponatraemia
B ketosis
C dehydration
D hyperglycaemia

Answers overleaf

77. C 14%

Alan will be dehydrated due to his polyuria. The dehydration will cause an increase in the pulse rate due to his decreased blood volume and a decrease in the blood pressure. Dehydration results in dry skin.

78. A 26%

In juvenile onset diabetes there is a breakdown of fat and protein in the body in an attempt to provide energy, therefore the child loses weight and feels hungry. The polyuria often leads to bedwetting in children and also to thirst.

79. C 69%

Alan is taught to be independent as early as possible and at 8 he is old enough to give his own insulin. However he still needs supervision and his mother needs to learn so she can give them if he is ill and unable to give his own.

80. B 56%

Because of insulin lack, glucose cannot enter the body cells to provide energy and the blood glucose level rises. In an attempt to provide the cells with energy body fats are broken down and converted to ketones by the liver, some of which are used by the body cells.
Excessive ketones accumulate in the blood stream which results in ketosis and acidosis causing the coma in hyperglycaemia.

James Stewart, aged 16 years, is admitted to your ward in an unconscious state. His general appearance was that of dehydration with deep sighing respirations and sweet smelling breath. A diagnosis of Diabetes Mellitus is made.

81. Which of the following is the reason for James' polyuria:

A an increased amount of antidiuretic hormone
B the osmotic pressure exerted by the glucose in the urine
C increased excretion of sodium
D increased fluid intake because of thirst

82. How many units in an insulin syringe, of 80 strength (80 units per ml) soluble insulin must be given for James to receive 24 units:

A 6 units
B 12 units
C 9 units
D 24 units

83. Which of the following is the *most* important when teaching James how to administer his insulin? That he should

A always vary the site
B be aware that insulin is available in different strengths
C dispose of the used needles and syringes safely
D give the injection at an angle

84. Which of the following indicate *early* symptoms of hypoglycaemia:

A hot, sweating, slow pulse
B fast pulse, dizziness, sweating
C blurred vision, confusion, disorientation
D hyperventilation, polyuria, palpitations

Answers overleaf

81. B 61%

When blood sugar rises above the renal threshold of 10 mmols/litre not all the glucose in the filtrate can be reabsorbed back into the blood and hence glucose appears in the urine. A large quantity of glucose in the urine increases the osmotic pressure in the filtrate which draws water from the capillaries into the tubule, resulting in polyuria.

82. A 83%

Number of units prescribed = 24 units
20 units per ml strength = 24 units in the insulin syringe
40 units per ml strength = 12 units in the insulin syringe
80 units per ml strength = 6 units in the insulin syringe

83. B 78%

All are important but B is vital because if James is given the wrong strength of insulin he could induce a hypo or hyperglycaemic state. After March 1983 only one strength of insulin will be generally available in order to reduce the risks of mistakes being made.

84. B 67%

This is due to the secretion of adrenaline (adrenaline mobilises liver glycogen when blood glucose levels are low) and results in tachycardia, tremor and sweating. As the brain is dependent on glucose also, a low blood glucose level leads to dizziness and abnormal behaviour prior to rapid loss of consciousness.

Mrs Wood, aged 38 years, was admitted to hospital for a partial thyroidectomy because of long standing thyrotoxicosis.

85. Which of the following pre-operative observations need to be reported immediately:

    A cardiac arrhythmia
    B heat intolerance
    C tachycardia
    D diarrhoea

86. Which of the following is the most likely after surgery:

    A transient swallowing difficulty
    B some disturbance of calcium metabolism
    C difficulty in adjusting emotionally
    D hypothyroidism and lethargy

87. Immediately following partial throidectomy the *most* dangerous complication is

    A tetany
    B myxoedema
    C haematoma
    D hoarseness

88. Immediately following partial thyroidectomy, a doctor should be summoned at once if you observe

    A cessation of drainage
    B pallor
    C high temperature
    D slow pulse

Answers overleaf

85. A 74%

One of the serious complications of thyrotoxicosis is the development of a cardiac arrhythmia. It should be reported immediately to prevent a life threatening situation. Distractors B, C and D are all to be expected when a patient has an overactive thyroid gland.

86. A 61%

Due to the position of the wound, swallowing may be difficult for a few days due to the localised trauma. Disturbance of calcium metabolism should not occur unless the parathyroid glands have been damaged or removed accidentally. There is no reason why Mrs Wood should not be able to adjust emotionally following the operation.
Hypothyroidism should not occur unless too much of the gland has been removed.

87. C 59%

Immediately after surgery haematoma is the ***most*** dangerous complication. Bleeding may occur post-operatively resulting in a haematoma under the clips or sutures. This can cause tracheal compression, choking and breathing difficulties. Please note, haemorrhage can occur and seep through the wound and trickle around to the back of the neck.
If no swelling beneath the wound is evident and the patient does not have pressure symptoms, then the clips will not be removed, for although bleeding has occurred there is no haematoma.
Tetany may occur if the parathyroid glands have been damaged or removed and the plasma level of calcium is low. Myxoedema may occur if too much of the thyroid gland has been removed.

88. C 43%

Drainage is usually minimal and cessation of drainage could occur. Pallor could be expected post-operatively.
A high temperature may indicate the onset of a thyrotoxic crisis and should be reported urgently as this is an emergency situation.
Thyroxine liberated from the gland during surgery will have increased the metabolic rate markedly resulting in tachycardia, pyrexia and restlessness. Cardiac arrhythmias and exhaustion may arise if not treated urgently.

Mr Smith, aged 52, is a metal worker and is myopic. Having removed his protective goggles for a few minutes he got a piece of metal in his left eye and so attends the Accident and Emergency Department for treatment.

89. A person with myopia

A is long sighted
B is short sighted
C has glaucoma
D has retinopathy

90. Why would fluorescine be instilled into the affected eye? In order to

A anaesthetize the eye
B wash out the metal fragment
C show corneal abrasions after removal of metal
D prevent bacterial infection

91. Which of the following would be carried out after Mr Smith's eye has been anaesthetized:

A his eye would be double padded
B the left eye would be padded
C the right eye would be padded
D he would be advised to wear dark glasses

92. In order to inspect the under surface of Mr Smith's upper eyelid it would be

A inverted
B everted
C retroverted
D circumverted

Answers overleaf

89. B 70%

Long sight is termed hypermetropia, glaucoma is raised intra-ocular pressure (i.e. in front of the lens), and retinopathy is a degenerative state e.g. diabetic retinopathy.

90. C 63%

Fluorescine drops stain the cornea an orange colour which, when examined closely, will highlight corneal abrasions. It is not an anaesthetic, douche or antiboitic eyedrop.

91. B 76%

It is necessary for Mr Smith to wear an eye pad on the affected eye after anaesthetizing it because should grit, dirt or some other foreign body touch the cornea, he would not feel it and a corneal ulcer would occur.

92. B 57%

Eversion of eyelid is the term used when the under surface of the lid is inspected.

Mrs Spock lives alone and has no previous hospital admissions. Following a cerebro vascular accident she has a dense right side hemiplegia and aphasia. On admission she is fully conscious although rather dazed and has urinary incontinence.

93. Which of the following is *most* likely to cause Mrs Spock great anxiety in the first 24 hours following admission:

A inability to move her right side
B fear of being in hospital for the first time
C being unable to communicate her needs
D the possibility of soiling her bed

94. Which of the following would help to maximise her feeling of independence during her first week in hospital:

A easy access to her locker and personal things at all times
B encouragement to participate whilst you bed-bath her
C cut up her food and ask her to feed herself
D dress her in her own clothes so that she can retain her identity

95. After 2 weeks Mrs Spock is beginning to regain some movements in her right leg. Which of the following objectives would it now be appropriate to incorporate into her care plan:

A stand and balance unaided within 2 days
B encourage active exercises to strengthen the leg
C walk with tripod unaided within 2 weeks
D stand with assistance and balance unaided within 1 week

96. Which of the following objectives is it most important for Mrs Spock to achieve prior to discharge to her own home:

A achieve full control of urinary bladder, speak appropriate phrases
B do her own housework, speak appropriate phrases
C dress independently, do her own housework
D achieve full control of urinary bladder, dress independently

Answers overleaf

93. C 60%

All of the problems stated are ones which will cause anxiety. However, within the first 24 hours Mrs Spock will be emotionally shocked and probably unable to comprehend the extent of her physical problems. Immediately following a stroke many people are unaware of their paralysed limbs, realisation tends to be a gradual process. Mrs Spock will be too overcome with the enormity of the situation to worry about the specific problem of being in hospital for the first time. Without communication Mrs Spock cannot adequately convey any of her fears and anxieties and this problem must therefore override all of the others.

94. A 41%

The question specifically asks what would maximise her *feeling* of independence. In all the distractors the nurse is actually doing some basic daily living activity for her i.e. cutting up her meal, dressing her, washing her, thus reinforcing her dependence. Only in A has Mrs Spock, the freedom to do what she pleases when she pleases.

95. D 41%

This question necessitates the student to first of all be able to recognise an objective and secondly to decide if it is a resonable one. The statement in A is an objective but for Mrs Spock totally unreasonable. With a dense hemiplegia it is highly unlikely that she will be able to balance in two days. The statement of B is not an objective but a nursing action. The objective in C is again unrealistic; it is very unlikely that she will be able to walk unaided within two weeks. D is the only answer which states a reasonable objective for Mrs Spock allowing for the fact that rate of recovery cannot be accurately predicted.

96. D 61%

Mrs Spock lives alone and therefore to some extent all of the items in the question are important, however you were asked to choose priorities. The answer is D because these are all activities which she must be able to cope with alone because even with supportive services there will be occasions when no-one is there to help her. The two distractors in the remaining alternatives which are less important for her to be able to do are i) speak appropriate phrases - there are alternatives to speech i.e. writing ii) do her own housework - a home help service can do this for her.

Sally Bowler, aged 8, is admitted apparently having had a grand mal epileptic fit. A family history was obtained from her parents and a chemical examination, blood profile, skull X-rays, lumbar puncture, EEG and brain scan were performed with negative results. Phenytoin 50 mgms three times daily and phenobarbitone 15 mgms twice a day were commenced.

97. Serum calcium levels will specifically aid diagnosis of

A cerebral tumour
B parathyroid dysfunction
C bone disease
D brain damage

98. Which of the following will predispose to gum hypertrophy in Sally's case:

A inadequate dental care
B inadequate calcium in the diet
C the effcct of phenobarbitone
D the effect of phenytoin

99. Which of the following will Sally be entitled to when she is 18 years old:

A free dental treatment
B free prescriptions
C child benefit
D attendance allowance

100. Which of the following describes post epileptic automatism:

A being unaware of actions
B momentary amnesia
C deep sleep
D post epileptic twitching

Answers overleaf

97. B 87%

Parathyroid dysfunction may lead to severe tetany as a result of hypoparathyroidism, and the subsequent altered calcium levels could give rise to convulsions. Serum calcium levels will ***specifically*** aid this diagnosis, hence B is correct.

98. D 52%

Gum hypertrophy in Sally's case is due to the side effect of phenytoin sodium.

99. B 61%

As Sally has a chronic disorder she will qualify for free prescriptions after the age of 18 years. She will then be too old to qualify for child benefit and it is unlikely that her epilepsy will be so severe that her parents can claim 12 or 24 hour attendance allowance.

100. A 43%

Post epileptic automatism can sometimes occur after the epileptic fit.
Although the patient may appear normal they can be unaware of their actions for some time. It is the last of the "stages" of an epileptic attack - aura
tonic
clonic
coma
sleep
post-epileptic automatism.

On admission Shirley, aged 8 months, is fretful, pyrexial and vomiting with temperature 38.5°C. A diagnosis of meningitis is made.

101. Which of the following *best* explains Shirley's reluctance to be handled:

A general toxic effects of infection
B insecurity due to strange surroundings
C pain and discomfort experienced on movement
D anxiety and fear following lumbar puncture

102. Why is Shirley admitted into a quiet, darkened, barrier nursing cubicle? To

A encourage sleep and protect from pathogenic organisms
B prevent spread of infection and reduce photophobia
C protect from pathogenic organisms and reduce photophobia
D encourage sleep and prevent spread of infection

103. Which of the following aspects of the nursing care plan is *most* important? That

A mobilisation is started gradually from admission to prevent complications
B living activities as described by Shirley's mum are continued
C nursing care is planned in order to reduce disturbance
D nursing care and observations are performed at times when sedation has had its optimum effect

104. Nose and throat swabs would be sent specifically for culture and sensitivity because

A the organism responsible could have spread from the throat via the middle ear
B the organism causing the meningitis could have spread to the nose and throat making it infectious
C this is routine screening for children admitted to a paediatric unit
D it is the only way in which sensitivity to the organism causing meningitis can be discovered

Answers overleaf

101. C 68%

In meningitis any movement stretches the inflamed meninges causing pain. Insecurity, anxiety and the effects of infection may all be relevant but option C ***best*** explains Shirley's reluctance to be handled.

102. B 67%

Meningitis could well be infectious and photophobia (dislike of light) is a common symptom. Until the causative organism is identified barrier nursing should be instituted and steps taken to relieve photophobia will help the child rest.

103. C 63%

In view of the fact that disturbance causes Shirley's distress C is the correct answer. D and B would be painful for her and sedation may or may not be used. Care (including observations) could not be limited solely to these periods.

104. A 69%

In babies an organism from the throat can effect the middle ear and from there to the meninges and this would be a reason for collecting swabs. Option C may be true but the question asked for the ***specific*** reason for collecting nose and throat swabs in Shirley's case.

Malcolm suffers from cerebral palsy and has frequent convulsions. He can feed himself with help and supervision and uses the toilet but must be taken regularly. His diagnosis is status epilepticus, however, he has stopped fitting on admission following anti-convulsants given by the General Practitioner.
His urinalysis shows protein ++ and ketones and he has vomited twice since admission

105. Which of the following potential problems should be given priority in your plan of care:

A urinary incontinence and further fitting
B risk of falling out of bed and inhaling vomit
C possible urinary tract infection and dehydration
D possible confusion and parental anxiety

106. Which of the following actions should be taken initially when Malcolm starts to fit:

A reassure the other patients quietly
B place a padded spatula between his teeth
C summon help and begin suction
D keep under constant observation and remove harmful objects

107. What is the significance of the ketones present in Malcolm's urine:

A lack of dietary intake has led to metabolic breakdown of fats
B pathogenic organisms are probably present in the urine
C dehydration and electrolyte imbalance has led to the production of waste matter
D his problems may herald an early onset of diabetes mellitus

108. Which of the following measures may best help alleviate the harm that Malcolm suffers due to his fits:

A a course of ECT
B institutionalised care
C a protective helmet
D curtailing his activities

Answers overleaf

105. B 51%

Malcolm is likely to fit again, in which case he is in danger of falling out of bed if safety precautions are not taken.
He has already vomited twice, therefore he may vomit again and could inhale vomitus. Both these possibilities need to be planned for, the use of cot sides and careful positioning and observation of the patient being an important part of the care plan. As safety is a factor, B is given priority.

106. D 82%

D is the correct answer as observation will aid diagnosis and alert the nurse to complications and removal of harmful objects will protect the patient. A and B are both dangerous whilst Malcolm is fitting and C does not positively help the situation.

107. A 64%

A is the correct answer as this is the physiological mechanism which has led to ketonuria. Malcolm will not have eaten for several hours and he is vomiting, therefore abnormal food breakdown would occur. Fats are incompletely metabolised in the absence of glucose and ketones are produced. (This process does not only occur in cases of hyperglycaemia.)

108. C 71%

C is the correct answer as this is a measure which may be employed in the case of patients who fit frequently and it does afford some protection. A, B and D are not likely to be effective.

LOCOMOTION

Mrs Jane Dobbs has suffered from collapse of her thoracic vertebrae,(10,11) due to degeneration. She has had surgery to fuse the bones together and is to be nursed in a plaster bed for at least twelve weeks.

109. Which of the following will prevent pressure sore development? The patient will need to be

A lifted out of the cast 2 hourly
B turned in both halves of the bed strapped together
C placed in the bath at least weekly
D have pressure relieving devices put inside the plaster cast

110. Why may paralytic ileus develop in the early care of Mrs Dodds in the plaster bed? Because of

A the change to the horizontal position
B pre-operative starvation
C the pain from the operation site
D the development of anorexia

111. Spinal fusion is carried out by

A pinning the vertebrae together
B tightening the joining ligaments
C inserting chips of bone between the vertebrae
D injecting a sclerosant around the vertebrae

112. Whilst in the plaster bed the morale of the patient can *best* be maintained by

A promoting independence and conversation
B suitable activities using appropriate aids
C sitting the patient upright twice daily
D encouraging many visitors at the same time

Answers overleaf

109. B 65%

To nurse a patient in a plaster bed, provision must be made to alter the position to shift the pressure which will cause tissue breakdown. The back portion of the bed is the part the patient lies on for most of the time, but at least twice a day the front which has been moulded to fit the patient is strapped over the body and the whole casing turned on its supporting base.
Other modern types of turning spinal bed may be used to ensure good alignment during the healing period.

110. A 38%

When a patient is suddenly forced to remain horizontal for a prolonged period physiological problems often arise such as slowing of the gastro-intestinal activity leading to paralytic ileus. This causes vomiting, abdominal distension and dehydration, needing the usual measures of naso-gastric aspiration and intravenous fluid administration until peristalsis returns to normal.

111. C 21%

Spinal fusion is carried out by taking chips of bone from a part of the patient, usually the ileum, inserting them between the roughened edges of the vertebrae. Haematoma formation occurs and callus forms to knit the vertebrae together and prevent the movement and pressure of the faulty bones which caused the patient pain and disability.

112. B 58%

Twelve weeks on a plaster bed in the horizontal position can be depressing and boring and could lead to emotional and mental problems. Initiative should be used to adapt aids such as mirrors well placed to allow the patient to see the activities in the environment, and book supports and angled spectacles to allow the patient to read comfortably. A succession of visitors rather than several at one time should be encouraged as it is difficult to keep looking from one to the other frequently while lying flat.

John, the 7 year old younger son of Mr and Mrs Sellers, has been knocked down by a car on his way to school, and sustained a simple (closed) fracture of the shaft of his left femur. You are a passer by at the scene of the accident and go to John's assistance.

113. He is lying still and is conscious but dazed. Your *first* action should be to

A lay John in the semi-prone position, to protect his airway
B cover John with a coat to keep him warm
C assess the extent of any obvious injury
D reassure John's mother that you can deal with the situation

114. The *most* likely treatment for this injury in a boy of John's age is

A fixed traction by a Thomas splint
B the application of a plaster cylinder to the limb
C to nurse John on Gallow's traction
D internal reduction of the fracture

115. Which of the following would be the *most* appropriate gift to bring John in hospital? A

A colouring book and crayons
B large bag of mixed sweets
C scale model of a racing car
D large circular jig-saw puzzle

116. Which of the following is the *most* effective way of minimising accidents involving children of John's age on their way to school:

A the school should instruct the children to follow the rules of "The Highway Code"
B ensure there is a School Crossing Patrol on busy roads outside schools
C encourage parents to walk to school, escorting their children in both directions
D alert motorists to the dangers of driving near schools when young children are about

Answers overleaf

113. C 56%

John's condition could be made worse by moving him. If he has any fractures, a closed fracture would be made into a compound one thus increasing the possibility of infection. Any haemorrhage should be dealt with as soon as possible. John is conscious and can protect his own airway so A is not necessary. Actions B and D would be performed after C.

114. A 59%

This is the appropriate method of immobilisation. Gallows traction is only used for very young children, plaster of paris would not effectively immobilise the fracture, and internal reduction would increase the possibility of osteomyelitis.

115. A 73%

This activity is the best of the options for a child confined to bed in hospital because John could colour the book without help if the nurses were busy, there would be no storage problems as there would be with the jig-saw. The racing car could run out of John's reach and sweets are bad for the teeth and lead to poor eating habits.

116. C 23%

A child of John's age who is out alone is always at risk of running onto the road in front of traffic. If he is accompanied by an adult who can supervise him, this risk is lessened.
The Schools Crossing Patrol will only be able to watch the children at certain points, not for the complete journey.

Mrs Jones, a 75 year old married lady, was referred to the orthopaedic consultant because of severe osteo-arthrosis of her left hip. She was a plump happy woman but was not able to walk very far because of the pain. The surgeon agreed to a total hip replacement, but explained that it would be approximately 4-6 months before a bed would be available.

117. **Which of the following is the best description of the changes in the joint due to osteoarthrosis:**

A articulating cartilage roughened and eroded, inflammation of synovial membrane, growth of osteophytes
B thickening of synovial membrane. excess synovial fluid, destruction of articulating cartilage
C articulating cartilage worn away, growth of osteophytes, appearance of cystic spaces beneath the bone surfaces
D bare bone endings, stretched ligaments causing deformity, loose bodies in the joint

118. **Whilst awaiting surgery the care of Mrs Jones is directed towards**

A preventing infectious diseases that may be associated with arthritis
B maintaining function of joints by reducing her weight
C preventing and correcting deformities by relieving pain
D resting joints by immobilisation followed by an increase in exercise to develop the supporting ligaments

119. **Which of the following is a specific post-operative complication of orthopaedic surgery:**

A thrombophlebitis
B osteoporosis
C contracture deformity
D fat embolism

120. **What is the most important advice to give on discharge:**

A wear lace up shoes
B sleep flat on her back
C elevate her leg for part of the day
D not to cross her legs

Answers overleaf

117. C 24%

Pathological changes include patchy degeneration and splitting of the articular cartilage with exposure of underlying bone. New bone is laid down at the edges of joints resulting in the formation of osteophytes (a small outgrowth of bone).
B applies to rheumatoid arthritis. A and D are a mixture of diseases affecting connective tissue.

118. B 66%

As Mrs Jones is an elderly lady an important aspect of rehabilitation after surgery is to ensure that she becomes mobile as soon as she is allowed to by medical staff in order to prevent joint stiffness, chest infections, pressure sores and other hazards of immobility.
By reducing Mrs Jones' weight the chances of successful rehabilitation are enhanced.

119. D 63%

In adults long bone contains yellow bone marrow which is mainly fat.
When a bone is broken fat globules are released into the blood from the fractured bone and may block a major blood vessel.
Thrombophlebitis is a blood clot in a vein with inflammation of the vessel lining. In osteoporosis the bone lacks in mineral salts and becomes thinner. A contracture is fibrosis of muscle causing deformity. Whilst A, B and C may arise, they are not directly associated with orthopaedic surgery and so D is the only ***specific*** complication.

120. D 74%

Abduction of the joint and dislocation of the hip is more likely to occur if the patient persistently crosses her legs, therefore D is the advice given on discharge.

Mrs James attends the clinic with her daughter Julie who is eighteen months old. She is diagnosed as having congenital dislocation of the left hip. Julie will be managed on an abduction frame for a week and then undergo surgery.

121. During examination, with the newborn baby lying on a flat surface, the nurse would suspect congenital dislocation of the hip if

A Ortolani's sign is present on the affected side
B Babinski's sign is absent on the affected side
C the asymmetrical tonic-neck reflex is absent
D Kernig's sign is present on the affected side

122. Whilst Julie is nursed on her abduction frame it is necessary to develop a plan of care which modifies usual

A bladder and bowel habits
B growth patterns and milestones
C hygiene needs and respiration
D methods of feeding, activities and play

123. The aim of immobilising the affected leg on a frame prior to further treatment is to

A abduct the affected leg to a 45° angle
B adduct the affected leg to a 45° angle
C adduct and flex the affected limb
D abduct and extend the affected limb

124. Julie has undergone surgery and now has a plaster cast enveloping her from waist to toes on both legs. Which of the following toys would be most suitable for Julie to play with:

A cuddly teddy bear
B string of beads
C building bricks
D "chatty" telephone

Answers overleaf

121. A 40%

This demonstrates limited abduction of the affected hip indicating that the head of the femur is not resting securely in the acetabulum. The asymmetrical tonic neck reflex is only present during the first few weeks of life in normal babies. Kernig's and Babinski's signs are not relevant.

122. D 70%

Bladder and bowel habits, growth patterns and milestones, hygiene needs and respiration must all be maintained whilst Julie is in hospital with as little modification as possible. The nearer the hospital routine and environment is to Julie's familiar home surroundings and routine the better, if minimal disturbance is to result to Julie and her family.
Because of her plaster cast and immobility Julie's activity, play and feeding methods ought to be modified. Play at the bedside must be emphasised and foodstuffs should be easily chewable and high in fibre due to her position (flat on her back).

123. A 45%

When the affected leg is abducted to a 45° angle the head of the femur is forced into the acetabulum and spasm of ligaments and muscles is reduced.
The other options are incorrect as they will not achieve the above.

124. D 35%

As Julie's movement is restricted, so too is her ability to continue social development. A "chatty" telephone will best help her communication skills and continue development bearing in mind that she is only 18 months old and cannot move freely.

A 45 year old woman is admitted to the gynaecological ward with a history of menorrhagia and stress incontinence. A vaginal hysterectomy is proposed.

125. Which of the following defines menorrhagia:

A normal blood loss at the time of the menstrual period
B excessive blood loss at the time of the menstrual period
C diminished blood loss at the time of the menstrual period
D excessive blood loss between the menstrual periods

126. Which of the following is the most likely cause of this lady's stress incontinence:

A the depressive state of the patient's illness
B lack of bladder tone
C increase in abdominal pressure
D prolapse of the anterior vaginal wall

127. Why is a catheter in situ post-operatively? To

A reduce the risk of infection
B allow time for local oedema to diminish
C prevent further stress incontinence
D promote healing of the local area

128. When may post-operative secondary haemorrhage occur? Between

A 8-11 days
B 3-5 days
C 36-48 hours
D up to 24 hours

Answers overleaf

125. B 74%

Normal blood loss is termed menstrual flow whilst diminished blood loss during the menstrual period is termed oligomenorrhoea. Excessive loss between periods is known as metrorrhagia and needs urgent medical investigation.

126. D 63%

As the anterior vaginal wall has prolapsed it will cause increased pressure on the bladder. When the lady coughs, sneezes or laughs and the pressure increases even more, she is likely to suffer from a small amount of urinary incontinence which is both embarrassing and worrying to her.

127. B 54%

There is usually some swelling and oedema of the surrounding areas due to trauma. If a catheter is not in situ, urinary output must be observed closely as retention of urine may occur due to the pressure and swelling obstructing the urethra.

128. A 61%

Secondary haemorrhage is always due to infection and it will take this long for infection to develop post-operatively.
Other types of haemorrhage are "primary" at the time or just after surgery and "reactionary" when the blood pressure increases up to 36 hours post-operatively and may dislodge a ligature.

Mrs Lesley Agar, aged 21 years, is admitted with acute lower abdominal pain. She has been married for six months and her husband works for an oil company. A laparotomy is performed on Lesley and acute gonococcal salpingitis is diagnosed.

129. Which is the most probable long term problem which may result from this situation:

A habitual abortion
B dysmenorrhoea
C infertility
D dyspareunia

130. With which of the following antibiotics will Lesley most probably be treated:

A tetracycline
B penicillin
C Amphotericin
D metronidazole (Flagyl)

131. Which of the following is the most important reason for Mr Agar to see the Consultant? To

A discuss the future problems Lesley may have
B trace contacts and commence any necessary treatment
C counsel him about the resumption of marital relations
D discuss the situation with regard to a future family

132. What specific nursing measures should be taken to limit the spread of this infection in the ward:

A none are necessary
B use of gloves whilst attending Lesley
C barrier nursing procedures
D specialised disposal of all excretion

Answers overleaf

129. C 78%

Gonococcal salpingitis is often bilateral. The infective process in the uterine tubes leads to adhesions and scar tissue completely blocking the tubes. The result of this would, of course, be infertility which is the correct answer. The three distractors are not related to salpingitis.

130. B 59%

Penicillin is the first drug of choice in the treatment of gonorrhoea. Tetracycline is a broad spectrum antibiotic and is not very effective against the gonococcus. Amphotericin B is used as an anti-fungal agent. Metronidazole is used for trichomonal vaginitis.

131. B 75%

In order to find the correct answer to this question it is important to remember that Mr Agar will almost certainly have gonorrhoea. It is no use at all treating Lesley if she then continues sexual relationships with her husband before he is healed. One or other partner will also have caught the infection from another source. The correct answer is therefore B. The other distractors are also important reasons why Mr Agar may see the consultant, but are of secondary importance to ensuring that both partners are treated and do not become re-infected or infect others in turn.

132. A 49%

Gonorrhoea is spread by direct contact and in Lesley's case, as she has gonococcal salpingitis, by sexual intercourse. No specific nursing measures are therefore required to limit the spread of infection.

Mrs Graham, aged 29, is in the gynaecology ward for bilateral salpingo-oophorectomy. She has an inoperable carcinoma of the breast but looks generally well, although rather obese. Mr and Mrs Graham have no children

133. Which of the following *must* Mrs Graham be made aware of as a result of the operation:

A she will become depressed as she cannot have children
B post operative chest infection may occur due to her obesity
C the operation may predispose to metastatic tumour spread
D she will experience symptoms due to an early menopause

134. The choice of operation is

A directly associated with her breast condition
B a normal sterilisation procedure
C unrelated to her breast condition
D a particularly safe sterilisation technique

135. Which of the following courses of action should be taken when Mrs Graham is upset by remarks made by another patient who considers being sterilised as "sinful":

A gently explain Mrs Graham's reasons to the other patient in privacy and comfort Mrs Graham
B comfort Mrs Graham, support her decision and engineer to keep the two apart
C ask them both into the office and discuss the whole situation openly
D reassure Mrs Graham, make her a cup of tea and complete the incident form

136. Mrs Graham's post-operative management *must* include

A wound care and early mobilisation
B hormone replacement and chest physiotherapy
C contraceptive advice and radiotherapy
D temperature observation and reducing diet

Answers overleaf

133. D 79%

The most important thing for Mrs Graham to be made aware of is that removal of her ovaries will produce symptoms of an early menopause. This is something which Mrs Graham may be entirely unaware of and it is important for her to recognise these symptoms as she may otherwise relate them wrongly to her breast condition.
Distractor A is an important consideration and one which Mr and Mrs Graham would probably have discussed. With an inoperable carcinoma she is likely to be more concerned with her own future than the fact that she cannot have children.
Distractor B is something for the nurses to be aware of rather than something Mrs Graham should have to worry about. C is untrue, the operation site is a long way from the site of the primary tumour and should not be disturbed by the operation.

134. A 68%

Breast tumours in young women can be oestrogen dependent. Removal of the ovaries will remove the source of this hormone and the cancer may regress. This operation is not a normal sterilization procedure; ovaries are not removed under normal circumstances.

135. B 73%

This is an important question and exemplifies a situation which can happen on a gynaecological ward. It is important that the answer chosen does not breach confidentiality and offers some means of ensuring that a similiar incident does not occur again.

136. A 59%

Wound care would be very important as obesity and malignant disease are both factors which may impair wound healing. Early mobilization is necessary to prevent chest infection and deep vein thrombosis which Mrs Graham may be more susceptible to due to her obesity and malignant condition. Hormone replacement is contra-indicated because breast cancer may be hormone dependent. Mrs Graham will be sterilized by the operation so contraceptive advice would not be necessary. Temperature observation may be useful but would not take priority over essential post-operative care. A reducing diet considering Mrs Graham's very unfortunate circumstances would seem unnecessary unless she herself considers it worthwhile.

THE SKIN

Mary, a fair haired 19 year old university student, visited the health centre who referred her to a dermatologist. Subsequently a diagnosis of psoriasis was made.

137. Which of the following described the appearance of Mary's skin:

A raised scaly lesions
B lesions present around major joints only
C circumscribed dull reddened lesions with silvery scales
D circumscribed reddened lesions that frequently bleed

138. Which treatment is most likely to have been ordered whilst Mary was in hospital:

A dithranol cream
B Betnovate cream
C coal tar cream
D zinc oxide cream

139. Which of the following is most likely to have exacerbated Mary's condition:

A anxiety about her examinations
B contact with infection
C using a different soap powder
D recent antibiotic treatment

140. Erythema is

A slight bruising
B superficial redness
C local swelling
D marked itching

Answers overleaf

137. C 67%

The appearance of psoriasis lesions is often the diagnostic tool. The silvery appearance of the plaques is characteristic of the disorder and can prove to be a disfiguring and distressing condition affecting the scalp, body and limbs but rarely, if ever, the face.

138. A 49%

Many forms of medication are used in psoriasis and today it is known that Dithranol cream has a good effect upon the lesions. It is important to apply the cream in the correct strength (only as prescribed) and to avoid contact with healthy skin as burning could occur.

139. A 75%

It is known that psoriasis has a "psychological" factor in its aetiology. B, C and D may all influence the skin in some way but are not specifically linked with psoriasis. C is most likely to cause contact dermatitis whilst B refers to pemphagus (a contagious skin disorder when staphylococcus aureus infects skin lesions). Psoriasis cannot be spread and is not infectious.

140. B 81%

Erythema refers to superficial redness of the skin. "Eryth" refers to the redness - think of erythrocytes (red cells) to help remind you.

Sharon Hallows, a 21 year old secretary, was on a caravan holiday with her husband when she had an accident whilst cooking a meal. This resulted in burns of the whole of her right arm and hand, and the right half of the front of her chest and abdomen. Sharon is right handed.

141. Which of the following indicates the percentage of skin surface burned:

A 9%
B 18%
C 25%
D 36%

142. Which of the following poses the greatest threat to Sharon's life during the first 48 hours after the accident:

A infection of the burned areas
B shock caused by pain
C loss of blood through haemorrhage
D loss of fluid and electrolytes

143. Which of the following will best encourage Sharon when she is anxious about her recovery:

A draw the curtains round Sharon's bed and reassure her that she will soon learn to use her left hand
B advise her that it is too early to tell how badly burned she is, but the doctors will do their best to help
C tell Sharon not to look on the bleak side, at least she did not burn both hands
D inform Sharon that plastic surgery can perform wonders these days

144. Much of the burned area has sustained third degree burns. When would transfer to a hospital nearer home be most likely:

A on the day after the accident
B five days after the accident
C two weeks after the accident
D two months after the accident

Answers overleaf

141. B 73%

The arm and hand is 9% of the body surface, half the chest and abdomen together are 9%, so the area burned is 18%.

142. D 80%

Sharon is not likely to lose enough blood to endanger her life. Infection will not pose a threat at this early stage, although it must be minimised to prevent problems later. Sharon will be in pain, but the threat to life at this stage will be from loss of fluid and electrolytes as plasma will exude through the burnt skin surface.

143. B 65%

It takes some time before the depth of the burn and the extent of scar formation and reconstructive surgery can be determined, and at this stage Sharon needs positive encouragement.

144. C 59%

After two weeks Sharon's general condition will have improved, but reconstructive surgery will not have started. When she is transferred, the doctors at her new hospital will be able to assess the situation and plan a course of action.

DIGESTION

Mr Young, aged 52 years, is a married man with a grown up family who live away from home. Following investigation he is admitted to the surgical ward for an abdominal-perineal excision of the rectum.

145. Which of the following will patients suffering from carcinoma of the colon often reveal? A history of

A constipation and flatus
B constipation and faecal impaction
C diarrhoea and melaena
D diarrhoea and constipation

146 Which of the following would take *priority* in the care of Mr Young on admission to hospital:

A recording of his pulse and blood pressure
B testing his urine for blood
C reassuring his wife and family
D discussing his operation and the site of the stoma

147. When completing the admission history from Mr Young it is *essential* to find out

A what housing and toilet facilities he has
B what his occupation is
C what his hobbies are
D whether he lives in a flat or a house

148. Whilst recording the blood pressure at 22.00 hours the junior nurse reports that his blood pressure is 95/60 mm Hg. As the senior nurse on duty, your *first* action would be to

A notify the night sister
B ask the junior nurse to check the recording in another half hour
C notify the doctor
D check the blood pressure recording

Answers overleaf

145. D 63%

Alteration in bowel habit is the commonest history given by the patient in relation to signs and symptoms of carcinoma of the colon. A, B and C have many other potential causes.

146. D 59%

Of the options given A and B occur for every admission, likewise C in total nursing care. However Mr Young's care ***must*** include a discussion of what the operation entails and what a stoma is if he is to be adequately prepared for the major surgery facing him.

147. A 70%

All of the options are important, but the ***most*** important is to establish what housing and toilet facilities he has at home prior to operation. This is in order to make arrangements for any alterations as early as possible. Remember that he will have a colostomy to cope with.

148. D 84%

Junior nurses may make mistakes when recording blood pressure so check the reading that the junior nurse has recorded and reported to you. If her figure is correct notify the night sister who will decide on further action.

Mrs Ferguson is a 36 year old lady with an acute exacerbation of ulcerative colitis. She is married to a schoolmaster and has two children. At present she is mobile, but undergoing medical treatment with parenteral nutrition and steroid therapy prior to surgery in two weeks time.

149. Which will be of particular clinical significance in her urine:

A ketones
B haematuria
C glycosuria
D urobilinogen

150. Which course of action would ensure that Mrs Ferguson was fully prepared psychologically before surgery? To

A ensure that she fully understands the operation
B tell her the surgeon is very good and will explain it to her
C talk to her and her husband so that they can both understand the operation and express any fears
D ask a patient to see her who has had the same operation

151. Which of the following courses of action should you take when Mrs Ferguson wishes to have her bowels open:

A give her a bed pan and ensure her comfort
B tell her she can use the nearby toilet
C tell her she must use a commode by the bed
D assist her to an area where she can use a commode in private

152. Which position should Mrs Ferguson adopt following the administration of a retention enema:

A sitting upright in a chair with her feet elevated
B in bed with the head elevated
C safely sitting on the commode
D in bed with the foot of the bed elevated

Answers overleaf

149. C 62%

Glycosuria is a manifestation of prolonged steroid therapy and this is related to the altered carbohydrate metabolism that occurs. Steroid therapy does not interfere with fat metabolism therefore there is no incomplete breakdown producing ketosis. Steroid therapy does not produce haematuria. There is no effect on the biliary system in a person on steroid therapy, therefore the urobilinogen would be present.

150. C 52%

Ensuring that she understood the operation is not adequate as much of her fear involves her feelings towards her husband and her future. Similarly B is not an acceptable approach. C reflects that thought has gone into dealing with her problems and fears and considers the whole picture.
It also confirms that telling is not the only means of communication, but reinforces the value of listening. D is vague and unreliable.

151. D 47%

A bed pan would show an inappropriate assessment of this relatively mobile young lady. One of the main fears and anxieties is the fear of unpleasant odour. This not only has an effect on the individual but also on the other patients, creating a socially unacceptable environment. In order to prevent this the nurse would not adopt C as a method of care. By adopting D we are protecting the patient totally and other patients in the ward. She will feel more dignified and independent. She will have privacy and the nurses can monitor exactly what is happening at each bowel action and record it correctly. Since the patient has an infusion in progress, B is unrealistic.

152. D 60%

The object of this procedure is to ensure the medication is held in the bowel for as long as possible. This enema is not an evacuant but one which will reduce the inflammatory process in the bowel.
Position D would ensure the maximum penetration of the retention enema to the area in which it was needed for a therapeutic effect.

Ann has been admitted to the Children's Ward with suspected cystic fibrosis.

153. Which of the following would indicate the possibility of cystic fibrosis:

A steatorrhoea
B redcurrant jelly stools
C strong smelling urine
D oliguria

154. Which of the following will confirm a diagnosis of cystic fibrosis:

A sweat test
B faecal fats
C duodenal biopsy
D xylose test

155. When is the best time to give pancreatic replacement preparations:

A before meals
B with meals
C after meals
D in between meals

156. Which of the following should be given to supplement Ann's diet:

A ferrous sulphate
B water soluble vitamins
C Ketovite
D fat soluble vitamins

Answers overleaf

153. A 71%

Cystic fibrosis is a disease which affects all exocrine glands including those of the pancreas. The pancreatic ducts become blocked with mucus, preventing the flow of pancreatic lipase into the duodenum. Pancreatic juice contains amylase, lipase and trypsinogen. As a result, there is incomplete digestion of fats and the faeces become offensice, fatty and bulky steatorrhoea.

154. A 73%

As the sweat glands have ducts (i.e. exocrine) they too are affected in cystic fibrosis and produce excessive amounts of sodium which is measured by a sweat test. This will confirm the diagnosis, for although faecal fats would indicate the degree of steatorrhoea, it is not likely to ***confirm*** the diagnosis for there are several possible causes of fatty faeces.

155. B 39%

Pancreatic replacement contains pancreatic enzymes needed for digestion of food; giving the enzymes before, after or in between meals would result in less food for the enzymes to act upon, thereby reducing their effectiveness.

156. D 43%

Fat soluble vitamins must be supplemented as fat digestion is incomplete due to lack of lipase from the pancreas.

Mr Pratt has a provisional diagnosis of diverticulitis and has suffered from chronic constipation most of his life. He cannot tolerate large amounts of fruit and vegetables.

157. Which of the following is a consequence of constipation:

A extra fluid is absorbed making the faeces difficult to pass
B the rate of peristalsis is affected by the bacterial activity in the bowel
C extra fluid enters the bowel causing diarrhoea
D the faeces in the colon stimulates intestinal hurry

158. Why does chronic constipation predispose to the development of diverticular disease? Because

A Mr Pratt will have had to strain to open his bowels
B the pressures inside the bowel will have been increased
C a long standing bowel infection irritates the bowel
D the bowel will not have been able to function properly for a long period

159. Which is the *best* way to help Mr Pratt when changing his sheet soiled by slight faecal incontinence? To

A tell him to let nurse know next time he needs to use the toilet so she can provide a bedpan
B inform him that cleaning his bed is all part of the job
C reassure him that he will soon feel better, and stop worrying
D advise him that this is common and when treatment starts he will improve

160. Which of the following should Mr Pratt be advised to include in his diet on discharge:

A four teacups of bran daily
B a large helping of vegetables daily
C eat wholemeal bread instead of white bread
D eat as much fruit as possible

Answers overleaf

157. A 48%

One of the functions of the colon is to absorb water, and the longer the faeces are in the bowel, the more water is absorbed.
Intestinal hurry usually refers to diarrhoea which is related to stress or anxiety.

158. B 61%

Most authorities agree that chronic constipation causes increased pressures in the bowel which predisposes to diverticulosis.
Eventually the inflammation of the diverticula will give rise to acute diarrhoea.

159. D 79%

Mr Pratt needs positive encouragement in this situation; even if a bed pan or commode is provided he may still be incontinent, and he is unlikely to stop worrying if C alone is given. He may feel less guilty if he thinks the nurse understands that he cannot help being incontinent, and will be a little reassured if he realises the problem will soon be resolved.

160. C 63%

Wholemeal bread contains significant amounts of fibre. Mr Pratt does not like fruit and vegetables very much. It is most unlikely that Mr Pratt would be able to tolerate large amounts of bran as it is fairly bland and unpalatable although this would certainly resolve his constipation.

Susan is 1 year old and the only child of a single Caucasian girl who is living in bed-sit accommodation. Susan's father, a West Indian, has deserted the family. She is found to be moderately anaemic, has failure to thrive and is diagnosed as having coeliac disease.

161. Susan's anaemia is likely to be due to

A sickle cell anaemia
B thalassaemia
C blood loss in stools
D folic acid deficiency

162. The diagnosis of coeliac disease is confirmed by

A sweat test
B xylose test
C jejunal biopsy
D fat balance

163. Susan has oedema of her lower limbs. This is caused by

A impaired venous return
B poor cardiac output
C hypernatraemia
D hypoproteinaemia

164. People with untreated coeliac disease are at increased risk from

A carcinoma of the bowel
B carcinoma of the stomach
C ulcerative colitis
D Crohn's disease

Answers overleaf

161. D 39%

There is poor absorption of folic acid and iron in untreated coeliac disease. She cannot have sickle cell anaemia with only one West Indian parent and thalassaemia occurs in families from Mediterranean countries.

162. C 50%

Although Susan may well have had all these tests in order to find the cause of her failure to thrive, the diagnosis of coeliac disease is made following a jejunal biopsy which will show the characteristic flat villi. Usually three biopsies are taken.
A gluten free diet is given after the first. Nine months later a second biopsy is taken which should show normal villi. The child is then given gluten for three months following which a third biopsy is taken. If the villi are flat on this occasion it is proof that it is the gluten which is causing the problem.

163. D 56%

The malabsorption also leads to poor absorption of amino acids which can lead to oedema. The body's ability to produce plasma proteins is impaired thus altering the osmotic pressure of the blood and preventing return of fluid from the tissues into the blood stream.

164. A 21%

In coeliac disease the villi of the intestinal wall undergo changes which, if untreated, may ultimately become malignant.

Sarah Helliwell, aged 17 years, is 1.55 metres tall and weighs 76 kg. Her doctor has advised Sarah to attend slimming classes because her obesity is caused by overeating.

165. Sarah's height and weight are

A height 5ft 2", weight 11st 13lbs
B height 5ft 8", weight 12st 12lbs
C height 4ft 10", weight 12st 4lbs
D height 4ft 8", weight 11st 7lbs

166. Which of the following is the *most* satisfactory outcome of Sarah's visits to the clinic:

A Sarah reached her correct height-weight ratio
B her mother realised that Sarah had been overeating
C other people at the clinic made friends with Sarah
D an improvement in Sarah's attitude towards food

167. After 4 weeks she becomes discouraged and talks about abandoning her efforts to lose weight. How can she best be encouraged to continue? By

A pointing out that she is still overweight and needs to lose more weight if she is to remain healthy
B telling Sarah that she has done very well so far and she should try to keep it up and lose more weight
C informing Sarah that it is usual to lose more weight in the first few weeks, but a smaller weekly loss will continue if she persists with the diet
D suggesting that Sarah buys a pretty dress in a smaller size so she will have some incentive to lose weight

168. What is the principle behind Sarah's reducing diet? To

A minimise her intake of fat in the diet
B eat less carbohydrate and more protein
C take in fewer calories than she is using for daily activities
D increase her metabolic rate and burn extra fat

Answers overleaf

165. A 43%

1 kg= 2.2 lbs
14 lbs= 1 stone
76kg x 2.2 = 167.2 lbs
167 ÷ 14= 11 stones 13 lbs

1.55 metres= 155 centimetres
1 inch= 2.5 centimetres
155 ÷ 2.5 = 62 inches
= 5 ft 2″

166. D 62%

If Sarah does not learn to eat to satisfy hunger and for no other reason such as to combat stress or because of boredom, she will soon gain weight again and will have a constant battle with her weight. Long term success will best be achieved by D.

167. C 40%

Sarah needs to be encouraged and educated at the same time. A is not encouraging, B does not educate Sarah and D might actually discourage her if she has a considerable amount of weight still to lose.

168. C 57%

The only way for Sarah to lose weight is to burn off more calories than she is taking so the body stores of fat are used to make up the deficit. The ratio between intake and expenditure of calories is the crucial point here.

Mr Heath, an 80 year old widower who is deaf, is admitted with inoperable carcinoma of the bowel which has spread to the peritoneum.

169. Which of the following defines the peritoneum:

A fibrous membrane supporting the abdominal organs
B fibrous membrane carrying blood vessels to the abdominal organs
C serous membrane lining the abdominal cavity
D serous membrane lining the abdominal cavity and covering the abdominal organs

170. After being in hospital for four months, Mr Heath's state pension is

A paid to the administrator
B collected by the medical social worker
C kept in the hospital safe
D reduced in amount

171. Communication will be more effective if the nurse

A speaks louder than usual
B writes everything down
C stands to the side of the unaffected ear and speaks directly into it
D uses a low pitched voice and stands in front of Mr Heath

172. The *most* effective means of achieving adequate pain relief is to ensure

A that analgesia is given as prescribed
B that analgesia is given prior to the recurrence of pain
C frequent reviews of Mr Heath's prescription sheet
D a daily review of Mr Heath's progress with medical staff

Answers overleaf

169. D 69%

The peritoneum is a delicate serous membrane which lines the abdominal and pelvic cavities and also covers the organs contained in them.

170. D 58%

After eight weeks the patient or a relative should notify the D.H.S.S. that he/she has been in hospital for that length of time and the amount of money received in the future would be reduced as long as the patient is in hospital. If the patient is unable to do this, the Medical Social Worker should be consulted.

171. D 70%

Most deaf patients learn by a natural instinct to lip read, therefore it is important to stand in front of the patient so he/she can see your face and lip movements. Many nurses believe that by raising the volume of their voice and therefore their pitch also, the patient will hear more. However, for many patients, their ability to hear high pitched notes is the first defect to occur.

172. B 56%

Adequate pain relief is a vital aspect of management when caring for a patient with inoperable carcinoma. The ***most*** effective method of pain relief is to prevent reoccurrence of pain by carefully judging when analgesia is needed ***before*** the patient experiences further pain, as well as attempting to keep the patient as alert and independent as possible.

Mr Young is admitted with jaundice and suspected carcinoma of the head of the pancreas.

173. Which of the following describes the blood supply of the liver:

A portal vein and hepatic vein
B portal artery and hepatic artery
C portal vein and hepatic artery
D portal artery and hepatic vein

174. Which of the following may be caused by carcinoma of the head of the pancreas:

A pre- hepatic jaundice
B post- hepatic jaundice
C hepatocellular jaundice
D haemolytic jaundice

175. Why is there delayed clotting time in obstructive jaundice? Because of

A lack of bile reaching intestine
B excessive heparin production
C liver damage
D high prothrombin levels

176. Which of the following vitamins would fail to be absorbed fully after pancreatectomy:

A K
B B_{12}
C C
D D

Answers overleaf

173. C 71%

The hepatic artery supplies oxygenated blood from the heart to the liver. After passing through the liver all blood passes to the hepatic vein for return to the heart. The portal vein carries blood from the mesentery, stomach, spleen, pancreas and intestines to the liver. There is no portal artery

174. B 50%

Post-hepatic or obstructive jaundice occurs when the biliary passages outside the liver are obstructed. Hepatocellular or hepatic jaundice occur when liver cells are not functioning correctly and bilirubin is not excreted. Pre-hepatic or haemolytic jaundice is caused by an increase in destruction of red blood cells.

175. A 30%

Vitamin K is a fat soluble vitamin which is not absorbed when bile is absent as in obstructive jaundice. This will result in a delay of the clotting time of the blood and therefore increase the risk of haemorrhage as vitamin K is the anti-haemorrhagic vitamin.
It is for this reason that vitamin K may be administered intramuscularly with the premedication and regular blood tests taken to determine prothrombin levels.

176. A 67%

The pancreas produces lipase which aids in the digestion of fats. Following pancreatectomy the fat soluble vitamin K will not be absorbed.

John Davies, a 32 y… , is admitted to the ward following a haematemesis. He w… he hospital 12 months previously undergoing medical trea… lcer.

177. Mr Davies was treated w… olinergic drugs during his previous hospitalisation. Si… of these drugs may be

A dry mouth, urinary retention, t… rdia
B nausea, vomiting, urinary reten…
C blurred vision, diarrhoea, tachycardia
D constipation, nausea, vomiting

178. Emotional stress may be a contributory factor to peptic ulcer formation because of

A increased activity of the sympathetic nervous system
B excessive stimulation of the parasympathetic nervous system
C increased secretion of hormone enterogastrone
D decreased secretion of hormone gastrin

179. According to Norton (1962), which factors are important when assessing a patient's risk of pressure sores:

A mobility, activity, mental condition
B personality, medical diagnosis, mobility
C mobility, mental condition, medical diagnosis
D activity, mobility, medical diagnosis

180. Mr Davies' serum potassium level of 5mEq per litre, is

A seriously above normal
B within normal range
C seriously below normal
D slightly below normal

Answers overleaf

17 A 35%

Anticholinergic dru ... action of acetylcholine, thereby inhibiting vagal stim ... ne possible side effects of this action are dry mouth, uri ... tion, tachycardia, blurred vision and constipation.

178. B

Stress causes xces ve stimulation of the parasympathetic nervous system. The vagus nerve stimulates the gastric glands to secrete more gastric juice. The sympathetic nervous system does not control secretion of gastric juice. The hormone enterogastrone slows down the stomach movements whereas the hormone gastrin stimulates the gastric glands to secrete gastric juice.

179. A 42%

With the Norton scale, mobility, activity and mental condition are highlighted as important factors towards assessing a patient's risk of pressure sores. Personality and medical diagnosis are not identified factors on this scale.

180. B 72%

The normal serum potassium level is in the range of 3.5 - 5.0 mEq/litre.

1. POINTS TO REMEMBER

Objective test examinations are intended to cover a large part of the syllabus, and it is unlikely that you will be able to answer all of the 60 questions easily. It is therefore wise to be prepared for the fact that there may be a small number of questions that you are unable to answer and you should not allow this to spoil your concentration during the examination.

Read the instructions ***carefully*** before you begin.

The time allocation of 1½ hours for a 60 item examination may seem generous, but it is intended as "thinking" time, enabling you to choose the correct answer after careful, reasoned thought. There is only ***one*** correct answer to each question, but if there seems to you to be more than one possible answer, then read the stem of the question again. There will be some information there to guide you. For example "Which one of the following is the ***most*** important" indicates that all four alternatives could be important but one has priority over the rest. Similarly, "Which one of the following must be reported immediately" suggests that all four alternatives may be significant and ought to be reported, but that one deserves ***immediate*** action.

Note that it is possible to alter your choice of answer but you ***cannot*** then revert to your original choice, so think carefully before making your decision.

2. MARKING THE COMPUTER SHEET

Only a Grade B (soft) pencil must be used.

Enter your candidate number like this:-

CANDIDATE NUMBER	0	2	7	1

Write your
CANDIDATE NUMBER
in the boxes provided
AND mark the same
figure in the column
below each box
Mark the number
thus: ***0 2 7 1***

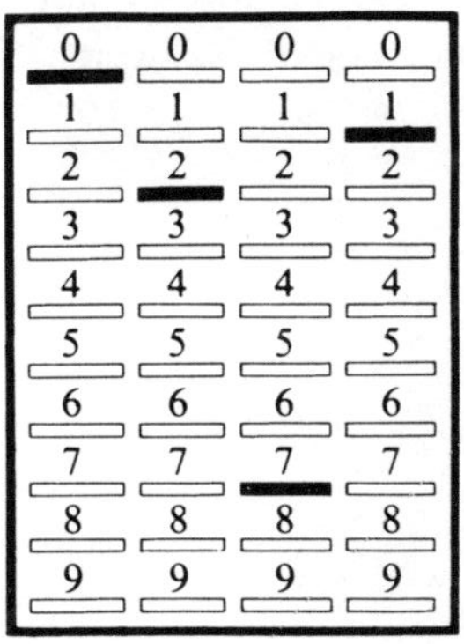

answering a question, mark the letter corresponding to the wer you consider to be correct. There is only one correct answer.

e.g. If you consider the answer to question 1 to be a) mark thus: using heavy pencil lines.

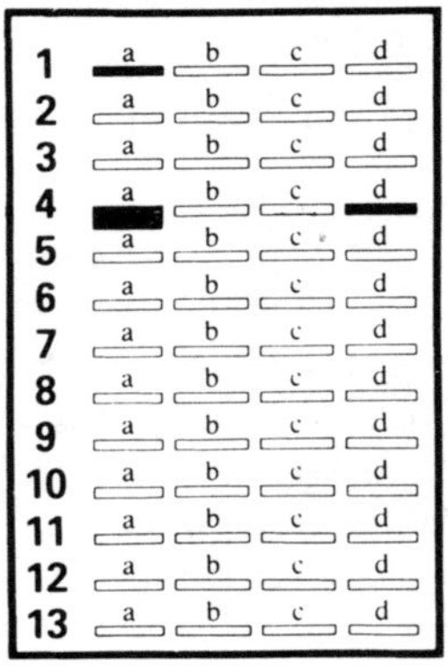

To cancel an answer fill in the bottom of the square thus: and re-mark the correct letter.

Do not use a rubber.
It is not possible in the case of question 4 to return to a) and re-mark it.

You should attempt all 60 questions as marks are not deducted for incorrect answers.

PRACTICE EXAM INSTRUCTIONS

This practice examination has been compiled, as far as possible, to correspond with the range of topics and degree of difficulty which one could expect to find in the SRN Final Examination.
Having completed the preceding 180 questions, you will be familiar with the "case study" format but the degree of difficulty of the practice examination falls within the range 24% - 80% and consists, as does the GNC State Final Examination, of case studies as well as individual questions, totalling 60 questions in all. The very difficult and very easy questions have been omitted in order to provide a realisitc examination.

There are 60 questions and the time allowed is 1½ hours.
Do not spend more than the allotted time.

Try to work under conditions which resemble those of the final examination. Do not refer to books, notes or speak to other persons.
Do not smoke - no smoking is allowed during the final examination.

Choose a time when you will be free from distraction and undisturbed, in a well-lit location. A watch or clock should be easily visible.

Answers, with explanations and degree of difficulty (facility value as a %) are to be found on page 108. The pass mark is 50%, i.e. 30 or more correct.

PRACTICE EXAMINATION

Susan age 6 years is the youngest of 3 children. Her father works as a labourer on a building site and her mother is 4 months pregnant. Susan has just been diagnosed as having cystic fibrosis, and has been admitted to hospital.

1. **Susan's symptoms are likely to include**

   A oedema and a low grade evening pyrexia
   B fatty stools and excessive perspiration
   C frequent chest infections and diarrhoea
   D failure to thrive and frequent chest infections

2. **Susan's disease will result in**

   A an inability to break down starch
   B a reduced intestinal surface area for absorption
   C a deficiency of pancreatic enzymes
   D a deficiency of bile salts

3 **Susan's siblings are very distressed at the separation. Her mother should be advised that they**

   A should not visit Susan as her sputum is infected
   B may visit Susan provided that they wear face masks
   C should be encouraged to spend all day on the ward
   D should visit for short periods of time on a regular basis

4. **Which of the following will be an important part of Susan's management:**

   A physiotherapy to her chest 2-3 times daily
   B antibiotics for the rest of her life
   C exclusion of all fat from her diet
   D special schooling in a pollution free environment

Mrs Walton weighs 80 kgs and is admitted for cholecystectomy and exploration of the common bile duct. She has a history of repeated attacks of cholecystitis and has been having a low-fat dict for six months.

5. The low-fat diet will include a reduction in her intake of

A scotch eggs
B wholemeal bread
C sugar on cornflakes
D lean beef steak

6. Why is a low-fat diet advised? Because

A pancreatic lipase has to emulsify and digest fats in the absence of bile
B the normal flow of bile would then be sufficient for digestion
C the gall stones would have a chance to resolve
D the incidence of infection leading to irritation of biliary epithelium is reduced

7. Prior to an intravenous cholangiogram it is necessary to tell Mrs Walton that she

A may feel uncomfortable when injected with the dye
B will be unaware of the test apart from the needle insertion
C may feel dizzy for 24 hours following the test and should rest quietly the next day
D will need to restrict her fat intake even more over the following 48 hours

8. Following surgery Mrs Walton will have a T-tube to

A drain the gall bladder bed
B direct gall stones into the drainage bag
C prevent adhesions of bile duct
D supply access for the cholangiogram

Mr Johnson, aged 75 years, is admitted to your ward with a chest infection and deep vein thrombosis in his left leg.

9. Whilst taking a nursing history you note that Mr Johnson is deaf. Should you

A write everything down for him
B take him to a side ward and speak loudly
C find out if he has a hearing aid
D ask his relatives any relevant questions

10. Why is it necessary to give Mr Johnson heparin by injection? Because it

A may cause gastric bleeding
B destroys the intrinsic factor in the stomach
C is destroyed by the gastric juice
D may cause duodenal bleeding

11. What is the purpose of giving Mr Johnson Menthol steam inhalations before physiotherapy. To

A stimulate free drainage from the respiratory passages
B dilate the respiratory passages
C liquify secretions in the respiratory tract
D stimulate production of secretions by goblet cells

12. A home help service would be provided for Mr Johnson on discharge

A free of charge by the Regional Health Authority
B free of charge by local government authority
C by the Regional Health Authority costed according to Mr Johnson's pension
D by Social Services costed according to Mr Johnson's means

Michael Jones, aged 24, is admitted with suspected meningitis, he is drowsy and when disturbed is irritable and confused. He is a well built man and a keen rugby player. Clinical examination revealed photophobia, neck rigidity, a positive Kernig's and Babinski's sign.

13. **A positive Babinski's sign is**

    A plantar flexion of the great toe
    B dorsal flexion of the great toe
    C resistance to extension of the knee
    D resistance to flexion of the knee

14. **Bacterial meningitis was suspected because of a nasal injury. Following a lumbar puncture you would expect the cerebrospinal fluid to contain**

    A increased protein, increased glucose
    B increased protein, decreased glucose
    C decreased protein, increased leucocytes
    D increased protein, decreased leucocytes

15. **Following a lumbar puncture it is most important to observe the patient's**

    A nasal discharge
    B pulse and blood pressure
    C temperature
    D level of consciousness

16. **Following culture and sensitivity being performed on the cerebrospinal fluid, Michael commences chloramphenicol. He should then have**

    A white cell count checked regularly
    B urine tests daily
    C a glass of milk with his injection
    D an increased fluid intake

Mr Adams, aged 53 years, is admitted for left nephrectomy following a history of problems related to renal calculi.

17. On return to the ward following straightforward left nephrectomy Mr Adams would have

A an intravenous infusion and urinary catheter
B a precautionary drain to kidney bed
C a naso-gastric tube and wound bed drain
D a urinary catheter on continuous drainage

18. Which statement is true in relation to the post-operative complication of paralytic ileus:

A the kidney is retro-peritoneal, therefore this is not a potential problem
B the peritoneum has not been opened, therefore this complication cannot occur
C as the retro-peritoneal area is disturbed this complication could occur
D due to the interference with muscles associated the diaphragm it would occur

19. Which of the following measures should be given priority in the post-operative period:

A chest physiotherapy
B leg exercises
C early mobilisation
D bladder irrigation

20. Which of the following observations will give most information about the functions of the kidney:

A temperature and fluid balance
B urine output and weight
C respirations and temperature
D urinalysis and fluid balance

Mr Grant, a 55 year old factory worker, has suffered from chronic bronchitis with emphysema for 15 years. He is admitted to your ward as an emergency with an acute exacerbation of his condition and is breathless, cyanosed and has a productive cough.

21. The characteristic dyspnoea on mild exertion is probably the result of

A lowered oxygen-carrying capacity of red blood cells
B impaired diffusion between the alveolar air and blood
C accumulation of mucus in the pleural space
D decreased tone of the diaphragm and intercostal muscles

22. Cyanosis is the result of

A increase in proportion of white to red blood cells
B decreased concentration of bicarbonate ion in the serum
C decreased diameter of peripheral arterioles and venules
D increase in the amount of reduced haemoglobin in skin capillaries

23. Mr Grant's sputum will most likely be

A thick and scanty
B white and frothy
C yellow and purulent
D blood stained and frothy

24. The nurse can help Mr Grant to expectorate more easily by ensuring he has an adequate amount of

A issues and sputum cartons
B nutritious diet
C fluids
D fresh air

Mrs Sally Watson, a 52 year old widow, is admitted for investigation of severe iron deficiency anaemia. The anaemia has caused three main problems, excessive fatigue, a sore mouth and dyspnoea on exertion.

25. What is Mrs Watson's blood test likely to reveal:

A hypochromic microcytic red blood cells and a haemoglobin level below 8 gm per dl.
B hypochromic macrocytic red blood cells and a haemoglobin level below 8 gm per dl.
C megaloblastic red cells and a haemoglobin level below 9 gm per dl.
D hyperchromic red cells and a haemoglobin level below 9 gm per dl.

26. Mrs Watson is distressed about the number of blood tests she is having. The nurse's initial action should be to

A explain why the tests are necessary
B check how many more tests are ordered
C ask the doctor to see her
D discuss Mrs Watson's anxieties with her

27. Why should the nurse administer the iron injection intramuscularly with a "Zig-Zag" technique?. Because this will

A reduce pain and swelling
B ensure the iron is rapidly absorbed
C ensure the iron is slowly absorbed
D reduce skin staining

28. Which of the following will help to ensure that Mrs Watson is motivated to complete her course of iron tablets following discharge?. She must understand that

A iron causes gastrointestinal upset
B she will not benefit from this therapy for two months
C iron must be taken with food
D oral iron causes temporary tooth discolouration

29. To evaluate nursing care, the nurse should

A collect information and identify any problems/needs the patient has
B assess the patient's response to the care and modify the care plan as necessary
C state goals towards which the nurses/patient can aim
D prescribe nursing care relevant to the identified problem

30. Which of the following are the most important principles of care following a total hip replacement:

A elevate the foot of the bed, keep the left leg adducted, pressure bandage to wound
B keep the left leg abducted, elevate the foot of the bed, pressure bandage to wound
C roll onto unaffected side for care, apply skin traction and abduct the leg
D roll onto affected side for care, apply skin traction and adduct the left leg

31. A patient appears to understand what is being said to her but cannot reply. Which of the following describes this type of aphasia:

A receptive
B jargon
C expressive
D sensory

32. Children who develop diabetes mellitus

A will always be insulin dependent
B can be managed on hypoglycaemic drugs in adult life
C are occasionally able to control their diabetes by diet
D require additional oral pancreatic enzymes

33. Indicate which of the following is the *most* effective way of preventing mistakes from occurring during the drug round:

A ensure all the patients are wearing their identi-bands
B make an example of any nurse who makes an error
C investigate any such episodes very carefully and record
D ensure nurses are familiar with the routine for administering medications

34. A patient is suffering from ulcerative colitis. The most important factor that the nurse should bear in mind when planning nurse care to deal with the problem of diarrhoea is to

A show the patient where the ward toilets are situated
B avoid milk and milk-based products
C make a list of foods not tolerated
D ask for a specimen of stool each day for inspection

35. Following a Ramstedt's operation it is especially important that care should include

A nursing in an incubator to maintain body temperature
B careful re-scheduling of feeds
C nursing with the head of the cot elevated to prevent vomiting
D aspiration of naso-gastric tube until bowel sounds return

36. Which of the following best differentiates between the pain of myocardial infarction and angina pectoris:

A pain following myocardial infarction is much more severe
B pain from angina pectoris is relieved by rest
C pain from myocardial infarction radiates down the arm
D pain from angina pectoris may be mistaken for indigestion

37. Immediately following a partial thyroidectomy the nurse observes a rise in temperature. She should

A observe the patient and perform ¼ hourly recordings
B tepid sponge the patient to lower the temperature gradually
C summon a doctor immediately
D inspect the wound for signs of infection

38. Following an above knee amputation which of the following complications may arise due to diabetes mellitus:

A flexion deformity
B phantom pains
C haemorrhage
D delayed healing

39. Which of the following would help the patient accept the fact that he has to have a below knee amputation? Explain to him that

A he will be free from pain once the leg has been amputated
B an amputation is the only treatment for an ischaemic foot
C rehabilitation care will be available for as long as he needs it
D an artificial limb will be fitted after the operation and he will walk again

40. A bleed into the anterior chamber of the eye is known as

A hyphaema
B hypopyon
C hypermetropia
D hydramnios

41. In order to facilitate removal of secretions when a patient has an acute chest infection, he is *best* nursed

A upright in bed
B in a supine position
C sitting out in a chair
D with postural drainage daily

42. Which of the following would be essential to help a newly discharged patient following an abdo-perineal resection:

A a letter to his General Practitioner
B Community Nurse to call within one week
C his follow-up appointment within 2 weeks
D the name of a patient who had the same operation

43. **Which of the following best describe the process of vomiting:**

A reflux of the stomach contents up the oesophagus against the peristalsic flow
B expulsion of stomach contents due to compression of stomach, relaxation of cardia and reverse peristalsis in stomach and oesophagus
C sudden emptying of stomach due to violent muscular contractions in stomach wall
D a feeling of fullness in the stomach associated with sweating and faintness that precedes the expulsion of food from the stomach

44. **Which side effects arise as a result of phenytoin sodium:**

A facial hirsutism and enlarged gums
B enlarged gums and alopecia
C opecia and pyorrhoea
D pyorrhoea and hirsutism

45. **Which of the following is a complication of chicken pox:**

A encephalitis
B vaccinia
C orchitis
D umbilicated vesicles

46. **Which of the following is the cause of the tissue changes which occur in rheumatic fever:**

A damage to body cells by micro-organisms
B excessive activity of polymorphonuclear leucocytes
C hypersensitivity of some immunity factor
D the absence of some immunity factor

47. **Which of the following are symptoms of salicylate intoxication:**

A tinnitus, sweating, bradycardia
B epigastric pain, sweating, liver damage
C epigastric pain, tinitus and restlessness
D vomiting, hypertension and restlessness

48. **Which of the following will the Guthrie Test detect:**

A dwarfism
B phenylketonuria
C lactosuria
D cretinism

49. **Which of the following would be the most appropriate time to administer post-operative analgesia and antiemetic. When the patient:**

A begins to look anxious and uncomfortable
B is fully conscious and vomits some bile stained fluid
C is alert and complains of pain
D has her hands and face washed several hours later

50. **Which of the following is the reason why a patient with nephrotic syndrome is susceptible to infection:**

A diseased lymphocytes
B decreased neutrophils
C reduced plasma proteins
D inability to produce antibodies

51. **One of the typical clinical features of trichomonal vaginitis is**

A frequency of micturition and dysuria
B greenish-yellow, frothy discharge and offensive smell
C whitish and thick copious discharge
D watery and whitish discharge with offensive smell

52. **The *most* common complication of an intra-uterine contraceptive device is**

A dyspareunia
B ectopic pregnancy
C spontaneous expulsion
D menorrhagia

53. Which of the following patients would cause you *most* concern. A patient, 24 hours following

A laparoscopy has slight distension of the abdomen
B vaginal surgery has a problem emptying her bladder
C abdominal hysterectomy is confused and pyrexial
D evacuation of uterus is still having some blood loss vaginally

54. Which of the following is thought to be an autoimmune condition:

A acute leukaemia
B Hodgkin's disease
C rheumatoid arthritis
D acute glomerular nephritis

55. Which of the following is a specific complication of vincristine:

A alopecia
B nausea
C constipation
D irritability

56. Whilst receiving a blood transfusion a patient develops tachycardia and hypotension. Should the nurse first of all

A inform the doctor
B increase frequency of observations
C stop the transfusion
D check for any pyrexia

57. Natural passive immunity is

A contracting the disease and recovering
B passed from mother to baby
C having a subclinical attack
D produced after vaccination

58. Which of the following is used without the need for a potassium supplement:

A Cyclopenthiazide
B Hydrochloriothiazide
C Frusemide
D Spironolactone

59. Which of the following would be the *first* course of action after a patient discovered his wedding ring was missing:

A institute a search of his locker and surrounding area
B remind him that the hospital does not accept responsibility
C reassure him that you will do everything possible to find the ring
D telephone the laundry to ask if a ring has been found in the dirty bed linen

60. A patient who has had a laparoscopy complains of abdominal distension the next morning. Which of the following is the *most* likely action:

A a doctor is requested to listen for bowel sounds
B the patient receives fluids only for a day
C two glycerine suppositories are given
D nothing as this is quite normal

<u>END OF PRACTICE EXAMINATION</u>

1. D 52%

There is a lack of pancreatic enzymes in this condition leading to steatorrhoea and failure to thrive. Mucus is excessively viscid and therefore is not expelled from the respiratory tract in the normal way leading to an increased number of chest infections.
There is unlikely to be a low grade evening pyrexia. When Susan gets a chest infection her temperature is likely to be raised throughout the day. These children do not sweat more than usual although their sweat contains an excess of sodium, therefore in hot weather they need added salt in their diet. There is no diarrhoea - the stools are bulky and fatty but not watery.

2. C 46%

The pancreatic ducts are blocked by the viscid mucus. This leads to a deficiency of pancreatic enzymes leading to poor digestion of fat and protein. Replacement enzymes are given with meals.
The intestinal surface area is unaffected. There is no deficiency of bile salts. The breakdown of starch commences in the mouth - salivary amylase.

3. D 51%

The siblings are younger and therefore long visits are inappropriate. Although Susan's sputum is infected she can be taught to cough into a pot or tissue. Face masks would be inappropriate and ineffective in protecting Susan. If one of the siblings developed an infection he/she should be discouraged from visiting until it had subsided.

4. A 54%

The aim of the treatment is to keep Susan as free from chest infections as possible. This is done by physiotherapy and encouraging Susan to expectorate the viscid mucus. Antibiotics are sometimes given for the first year of life but after that should be reserved for treating infections. Children with cystic fibrosis vary in their tolerance of fat; some manage with an almost normal fat content while others require a low fat diet. These children should live as normal a life as possible and Susan should be able to go to a normal school.

5. A 63%

Scotch eggs (eggs surrounded with sausagemeat) contain cholesterol, therefore their intake should be reduced. B and C do not require bile for digestion as they are carbohydrate; nor does D as it is mainly protein.

6. B 38%

Lipase depends on bile to emulsify fats - it cannot perform this function itself. If fat intake is reduced, stored bile is not required and the gall bladder will not be called on to contract. This could lead to expulsion of a stone into the cystic duct. Bile production itself is reduced if less fat is ingested hence reducing the amount directed to the gall bladder. There is no evidence that gall stones will dissolve naturally once formed and irritation of the epithelium precedes infection.

7. A 24%

A hot, burning sensation over the body is common during injection of the dye. She may feel A and should be prepared, although she should not have any ill effects after the tests and should seek advice if she feels unwell. The dye has no effect on bile function.

8. C 29%

The common bile duct has been explored leading to inflammation of the epithelial lining - adhesions could occur if the lining is not kept separate. A separate drain is used for the gall bladder bed. D is not the ***reason*** for inserting the t-tube but is often used for this purpose 7 - 10 days post-operatively.

9. C 76%

Find out if he has a hearing aid - if so it will be much easier for both of you. If he does not have one then sit down with him and ensure you are at the same level. Face him and speak slowly and clearly. B would be ineffective and A and D are innappropriate at this early stage although may perhaps be considered later.

10. C 62%

Heparin is a protein substance and if given by mouth it would be rendered inactive as the pepsin in the gastric juice would start to digest it.

11. C 65%

By breathing steam Mr Johnson is inhaling warm, moist air into the respiratory passages which helps to make the mucus lining the air passages less viscid and therefore easier to expectorate.

12. D 57%

Home helps are provided by the Social Services but the patient/client is asked to make a contribution to her wages and this is based on how much the patient/client can afford to pay.

13. B 31%

Normally when the sole of the foot is stroked lightly the toes will curl downwards but if Babinski's sign is positive the big toe bends upwards indicating abnormality.
Options C and D relate to Kernig's sign.

14. B 24%

Because of the bacterial infection of the cerebro-spinal fluid the normal glucose content is lowered as the bacteria use some of the glucose for their own nutrition. Similarly as a result of the infection the protein level will rise as part of the body's defence system.

15. D 73%

If the patient has raised intra-cranial pressure removal of the cerebro-spinal fluid during a lumbar puncture could possibly result in "coning" and increased pressure on the brain stem. Consequently the patient will become increasingly drowsy.

16. A 43%

Granulocytes are white blood cells and agranulocytosis (a reduction in the number of granulocytes) is a side effect of chloramphenicol so a regular white cell count is important. The granulocytes play a major part in body defences and an early symptom of agranulocytosis is an infected sore throat.

17. B 28%

All the other distractors contain unnecessary post-operative measures.
Urinary catheter is not required as urine should continue to be secreted by the remaining kidney. There is no reason to pass a naso-gastric tube unless gastro-intestinal complications occur.
The presence of a catheter will also add the risk of urinary tract infection which would be particularly undesirable because of the risk of ascending infection to the remaining kidney.

18. C 63%

The fact that the retro-peritoneal area is disturbed means that the adjacent bowel will also be handled thus increasing the risk of paralytic ileus occurring post-operatively. The interference with the diaphragm would not affect the peristaltic action of the ileum.

19. A 39%

The question asks for the priority measures, it does not imply that other measures are unimportant. The position of the wound will mean that lung expansion is painful and difficult; the resulting shallow respiratory movements will increase the risk of Mr Adams developing a post-operative chest infection. Leg exercises would be necessary but there is no indication that Mr Adams is at any increased risk of a deep vein thrombosis.

20. D 63%

Information about the right kidney i.e. the remaining kidney is required. Urinalysis changes commonly occur in renal disease. Fluid balance obviously reflects the ability of the kidney to adjust output in relation to fluid intake. Temperature changes do not reflect any changes in kidney function. Urine output is useful but only in relation to the input. Weight may also be useful but only if oedema is present.

21. B 79%

Because of Mr Grant's emphysema coupled with his acute exacerbation of already existing bronchitis, the surface area of lung tissue available for diffusion of oxygen between alveolar air and blood capillaries surrounding the alveoli, is reduced. A, C and D are not relevant.

22. D 55%

Cyanosis is always associated with oxygen lack. In Mr Grant's case there is impaired diffusion of oxygen into red cells therefore some haemoglobin remains unaltered instead of becoming oxyhaemoglobin the red cells pass through the pulmonary vessels.

23. C 35%

Mr Grant has a superimposed acute chest infection in addition to his chronic bronchitis, therefore his sputum will be yellow and purulent as a result of the infective processes.

24. C 60%

If Mr Grant is pyrexial and sweating he is likely to become easily dehydrated. Should this occur, fluid in the respiratory secretions will be reabsorbed making sputum thick, tenacious and difficult to expectorate. Prevention of dehydration will indirectly help Mr Grant expectorate more easily.

25. A 48%

Small (microcytic) and pale (hypochromic) red cells are produced in iron deficiency anaemia and a haemoglobin of less than 8 gm/dl would produce Mrs Watson's symptoms. Macrocytic, megaloblastic (large immature cells) anaemia results from B_{12} deficiency.

26. D 63%

Initially it would be best to sit and talk to Mrs Watson about her anxiety although A, B and C are all possibilities later.

27. D 77%

The "zig-zag" route prevents iron back tracking up the injection track which would lead to skin staining.

28. B 42%

Mrs Watson will need to understand about the delayed effect of therapy or she may decide that the tablets are useless and discontinue treatment. Additionally she will need to be told of the discoloured stools and possibility of gastric upset - however, B is the alternative which she ***must*** understand in order to encourage her to complete the course of tablets.

29. B 57%

This question ***refers*** to stages of the process of nursing.
Option A describes stage 1 - assessment of the patient's needs and problems.
Option C describes stage 2 - stating goals or anticipated outcomes of the care to be given.
Option D describes stage 2 also - planning or prescribing the nursing care needed by the patient in order to meet the needs or alleviate the individual problems highlighted on assessment. Option B summarises stage 4 - that of evaluating care given and modifying nursing plans as appropriate.
Stage 3, actually giving care to the patient, or helping the patient and/or family to give care completes the 4 stages of the nursing process although not referred to in any of the options of this particular question.

30. B 58%

The aim of care is to ensure the head of the femur is firmly embedded in the acetabulum which will be achieved by the actions in B. Adduction, rolling the patient instead of lifting up in the horizontal position and skin traction would achieve the opposite effect.

31. C 46%

Aphasia is a defect or loss of the power of expression by speech, writing or signs, or of comprehending spoken or written language due to injury or disease of the brain centres.
Expressive aphasia is that in which the patient understands what is being said and knows what to say in reply, but cannot utter the words.
Receptive and sensory aphasia both describe the situation where the patient cannot understand the written or spoken word.
Jargon aphasia consists of meaningless words and phrases spoken by the patient.

32. A 78%

Children who develop diabetes mellitus are insulin dependent.
If they have insufficient insulin production from the Islets of Langerhans in childhood they are not going to manage on hypoglycaemic drugs alone in later life or control their diabetes by diet alone for patients able to do this do have some insulin being produced naturally by their pancreas. Oral pancreatic enzymes will be of no value - insulin is a hormone.

33. D 73%

If the correct routine is always followed, mistakes are less likely to happen. Answer A is only effective if the nurses always check the identibands before administering medicines. Education of awareness of potential problems is more effective than investigation and personal degradation after the incident.

34. C 45%

The toilets may be occupied, the need to defaecate is very urgent and there may not even be time to reach the toilet. If bowel movements are very frequent all specimens need to be inspected and charted. Some patients do find milk an irritant but this is not a 'routine' taboo in all regimes. All stools need to be examined, not just one specimen daily, therefore the way to minimise the problem of diarrhoea is to ensure that irritating foods are noted and avoided.

35. B 26%

In a Ramstedt's operation the pyloric muscle is split, the gastric mucosa is left intact. It is important that post-operative feeds are carefully increased; the amount and strength should not be increased at the same time. There is no reason why the baby should not be able to maintain his own temperature in a warm ward.
An incubator will make his mother feel that he is iller than he in fact is.
It is unlikely that C will prevent vomiting in this case.
It is important that the baby is positioned carefully so that if he does vomit he will not inhale; these babies are usually nursed flat in the lateral or prone position. The intestines have not been handled so there should be no interruption to bowel sounds.

36. B 58%

The main feature of pain following myocardial infarction is that it is constant. Again pain may be severe and answers C and D apply equally to both types of pain. Only the pain of angina is relieved by rest when oxygen supply to the myocardium increases as exercise is stopped.

37. C 41%

A rise in temperature ***immediately*** following partial thyroidectomy indicates that the patient may be undergoing a thyroid crisis and this is a medical emergency. Thyroxine is released into the blood stream when the gland is handled during surgery. The metabolic rate is increased and consequently the patient becomes hyperpyrexial, has tachycardia and may become exhausted and develop heart failure if urgent treatment is not given.

38. D 80%

All the options are complications following above knee amputation on any patient. However, diabetic patients are more liable to have delayed healing due to their diabetic condition. A diabetic patient is also more liable to infection.

39. C 32%

The patient following an amputation may require varying time periods to be able to manage again. Therefore rehabilitation is designed to suit the patient and his problems. It is very important that the patient understands this and does not feel he will be left to manage alone. Although the patient will not experience the same pain following amputation he may experience phantom pains which result from the cutting of nerve fibres during operation. These pains will subside over a period of time and do not require analgesia.

40. A 56%

A hyphaema is a bleed into the anterior chamber of the eye i.e. in front of the pupil. Because of this the blood occludes part of the pupil and can be easily distinguished. A hypopyon is a stye, hypermetropia is long sight and hydramnios is excessive amniotic fluid around a foetus.

41. D 51%

B is obviously incorrect - a patient with a chest infection is not best nursed flat on his back. Of the other three alternatives, A and C will help by facilitating lung expansion but D provides the ***best*** answer. Postural drainage daily will help drain secretions out of the lungs and expectoration will be easier.

42. B 73%

All four alternatives may be of some help to a newly discharged patient with a colostomy, but of most value would be a visit from the community nurse as she could assess the patient's ability to cope at home, as well as answer his immediate queries/worries related to the stoma.

43. B 28%

All distractors partly describe the process of vomiting but B is the ***best*** description - which was asked for in the stem of the question.

44. A 33%

Many drugs have side effects and it is important to know those the patient may suffer, especially those likely to cause anxiety and embarrassment as well as discomfort. Phenytoin sodium may well cause gum hypertrophy and slight facial hirsutism.

45. A 20%

The chicken pox virus may cause inflammation of brain tissue i.e. encephalitis. Vaccinia is a localised pustular eruption produced by innoculation of the vaccinia virus, used to produce antibodies against smallpox. Orchitis is inflammation of the testes, is found in 25% of men and adolescent boys with mumps. In 83% of cases only one testicle is involved. Umbilicated vesicles are the lesions of ***smallpox*** which may develop into pustules, which exhibit a depressed area in the centre.

46. D 25%

Some absence of immunity factor is thought to cause the tissue changes of rheumatic fever. Infection is due to Beta haemolytic streptococcus and commonly affects children who do not effectively produce antibodies.

47. C 42%

Aspirin overdose causes epigastic pain, vomiting, hypotension, tachycardia, restlessness and disturbances in acid base balance causing hyperventilation. Tinnitus and visual disturbances may also be present.

48. B 78%

A Guthrie test is a heel prick in order to obtain blood for estimation of the amino acid phenlyalanine levels. If they are increased the body has phenylketonuria which is lack of the liver enzyme needed so that phenylalanine can be metabolised. If absent the levels of phenylalanine build up in the blood and are responsible for toxic brain damage.

49. A 63%

An anti-emetic could be given if prescribed when the patient vomits bile stained fluid. Post-operative analgesia may possibly be administered when the patient complains of pain or later, when making the patient comfortable if movement makes her pain worse. The question however, asked which of the four options was the ***most*** appropriate time to administer analgesia and anti-emetics. If the patient began to look anxious and uncomfortable post-operatively it would alert the observant nurse to the fact that pain may just be beginning or that nausea was preceding a vomiting bout hence it would be appropriate to give analgesia and anti-emetics then as prescribed.

50. C 44%

Proteinuria occurs in nephrotic syndrome, consequently the amount of circulating plasma proteins is diminished (including globulin). As globulin plays an important part in body defences a patient with a deficiency of plasma proteins is susceptible to infection.

51. B 60%

Greenish-yellow frothy discharge from the vagina is a characteristic feature of trichomonas vaginitis and is caused by the protozoa which is responsible for the infection.

52. D 71%

Menorrhagia (excessive blood loss at the time of menstruation) is the most common complication of an intra-uterine device, especially if fitted to women who have not had children.
Dyspareunia is painful or difficult coitus, an ectopic pregnancy is one in which the foetus is embedded outside the uterus (commonly in the fallopian tube).

53. C 66%

Of the four options only C would be considered a serious post-operative state. A and D can be anticipated and the patient reassured by caring explanations that the condition will soon resolve. B may necessitate action by the nurse in order to help the patient pass urine, but C indicates that medical treatment is needed quickly and should cause most concern to nursing staff. Confusion and pyrexia should not normally be part of any patient's post-operative recovery period.

54. C 75%

Only rheumatoid arthritis is considered to be an auto-immune condition whereby the body's defences are directed against the body's own tissue resulting in inflammation and degeneration of joints.
Acute leukaemia and Hodgkin's disease are both malignant disorders.
Acute glomerular nephritis arises as a result of an allergic response in the kidney to the toxins of the Beta haemolytic streptococcus.

55. C 36%

Cytotoxic drugs have many side effects including alopecia, nausea and irritability, but these are not particularly specific in relation to Vincristine.
Gastric motility is slowed down by Vincristine resulting in constipation, hence C is a specific complication.

56. C 67%

The complications which may arise during a blood transfusion include i) agglutination of red cells, haematuria, loin pain, oliguria and acute renal failure ii) overloading of the circulation, distended neck veins, pulmonary oedema, dyspnoea and heart failure iii) allergic reaction to the transfused blood in sensitive individuals, progressing in severe cases to anaphylactic shock.
If a patient develops hypotension and tachycardia iii) above is likely, therefore in order to minimise the allergic reaction the blood transfusion must first of all be stopped, although A, B and C will also be necessary.

57. B 74%

Natural immunity means that the antibody formation has been stimulated in response to contact with the disease, whilst "passive" immunity means that the antibodies have not been produced inresponse to a specific infection but have passively been given to the recipient. Only B is passive, because the ***mother*** produced the antibodies which were then transmitted via the placenta to the fetus - the baby did not actively produce the antibodies himself. A is natural active immunity, C is natural active immunity, D is artificial or acquired active immunity.

58. D 63%

Only Spironalactone is used without the need for a potassium supplement. The others may lead to hypokalaemia because of excessive potassium excretion in the urine.

59. C 54%

The ring is quite likely to be found, and at this stage reassurance is in order, before the search is started. Although the hospital does not accept responsibility for patients belongings, this is not an appropriate time to remind the patient of this.

60. D 52%

After a laparoscopy the patient may well complain of abdominal distension - this is to be expected, therefore no action is necessary.